P9-DMY-227

Acknowledgments

Many thanks to Robert Diforio, our literary agent,
and everyone at Adams Media.

contents

Introduction:
The Ins and Outs of Detox

DETOX DIETS ARE ONE OF THE HOTTEST NEW TRENDS IN HOLLYWOOD. Popular in the 1970s, they are enjoying a renaissance among actresses, supermodels, and other celebrities, who are using them as fast-track methods for blasting fat and unwanted pounds in preparation for red carpet events and to restore equilibrium to bodies thrown out of balance by the stress and hustle of jet-set living.

Beyoncé made the Master Cleanse diet a household name, consuming nothing but jacked-up lemonade for 10 to 14 days to lose 20 pounds, while Anne Hathaway resorted to a 48-hour detox diet that also revolved around a lemonade mix. Gwyneth Paltrow embarks on a one-week cleanse a few times a year to feel lighter, eliminating dairy, caffeine, and processed food from her diet and eating only fruit-and-vegetable juices and soups and sugar- and soy-free meals. *Transformers* star Megan Fox cleanses her body and system with apple-cider vinegar and water. Other stars who swear by detox diets include supermodel Gisele Bündchen, fashion designer Stella McCartney, and Madonna. But if celebrities and supermodels are sold on detox diets, especially celebrity-style detox diets that encourage semi-starvation, the traditional medical community is anything but.

Maybe Beyoncé and Britney have gone on ultralow-calorie detox diets and lived to talk to about them, but unlike the rest of us, most celebrities have teams of medical specialists on 24-7 speed dial, in case their detox regimens go awry.

But are detox diets the answer for you? If you're confused about the conflicting information and have been looking for a nutritious, healthy, and medically approved way to detox, you've come to the right place. Whether you want to shed excess pounds, lower your cholesterol, cleanse your internal organs, or reduce your risk of serious diseases like cancer and diabetes, the detox diets, recipes, and meal plans in this book will help you achieve your health or weight-loss goal without forcing you to starve, spend the rest of your life on a treadmill, or engage in dangerous "purging" or "cleansing" methods.

Detox for the Rest of Us offers fifteen different healthy detox plans, ranging from 3-day to 30-day programs that encompass the full range of detox options, including juice detox, vegan detox diets, cholesterol detox, low-carb diets, low-sodium diets, and exclusion diets that remove common culprits like gluten and lactose from dietary regimens.

But perhaps the biggest difference between these detox diets and the others is that they are delicious and filling as well as safe and effective, combining proven detox foods in scrumptious recipes and meal plans that will satisfy your taste buds and appetite while helping you accomplish your detox goal.

The Best Detox Foods

- Apples
- Avocadoes
- Bananas
- Beans
- Blueberries
- Citrus fruits
- Dark chocolate
- Cruciferous vegetables
- Fish (cold-water)
- Garlic
- Ginger
- Green tea
- Nuts and seeds
- Oats
- Olive Oil
- Sweet Potatoes
- Tofu
- Quinoa
- Walnuts
- Yogurt
- Leafy Greens

Do You Really Need to Detox?

The body is under constant assault from toxins such as smog, pesticides, artificial sweeteners, sugar, processed foods, and alcohol. Your body usually does an excellent job of filtering out most toxins so they don't cause illness or disease. But when your immune system is compromised through illness, a poor diet, or negative lifestyle habits like excessive smoking, drinking, or drug use, your body may not be able to keep up with the damage. Without periodic cleansings in the form of detox diets, these poisons can accumulate in the body and cause headaches, fatigue, and a variety of chronic diseases. When done correctly, detox diets can support the body's natural process of detoxification.

Considering the efficiency of your own inner machinery, you might be wondering if you really need a detox diet. If you live a serene life in a monastery that's far from pollutants, the answer may be no. But if, like most people, you lead a hectic, stressful life that leaves little or no time for relaxation or exercise; you eat a less-than-healthy diet that often includes on-the-run fast and convenience foods; you don't get enough exercise; you overuse caffeine, alcohol, or drugs; and you rarely get enough sleep, you may be an excellent candidate for a detox diet. Pick a time to detox in which you are not facing major deadlines or have an especially packed schedule, as the stress on your body may be too great. Entering into your detox with a relaxed frame of mind will help you reap the most benefits from your effort!

Are You Entering the Toxic Zone?

Although modern medical science has a test for practically every disease and condition, they've yet to devise a foolproof test that determines whether or not you need to detox. To help you decide if detox is right for you, we have devised an easy, fun quiz that will help you target some of the more common diet and lifestyle habits that may be sending your system into toxic overload. Give yourself one point for every question you answer "yes," then follow scoring directions below.

1. I put salt on everything before tasting it.
2. I can get only one leg into last year's bikini.
3. I fall asleep to freeway traffic, electric static from overhead power cables, and/or the drone of circling planes.
4. Smoke gets in my eyes (lungs, hair, and clothing) from my cigarettes, or from the second-hand smoke of friends who smoke in my environment.
5. I use caffeine and other stimulants to stay alert and energized.
6. I'm either constipated or going all the time.
7. I abuse alcohol and drugs on a regular basis.
8. Anything with dairy or gluten in it leaves me . . . very quickly.

> **DETOX TIP**
>
> The body already has several systems in place—including the liver, kidneys, and gastrointestinal tract, which work together to eliminate toxins from the body within hours of consumption.

9. Some days I feel like a water balloon.
10. If I'm not glued to the computer, I'm on my BlackBerry, iPod, or cell phone.

Scoring Directions

0: Congratulations! You are living a healthy lifestyle that is free of toxins.

1–3: You're approaching the Toxic Zone. Your lifestyle habits may need some fine-tuning to avoid toxicity.

4–9: You've entered the Toxic Zone and will benefit from one of the fifteen detox diets in this book. See the helpful guide below for information on how to match your symptoms to the right detox diet.

10: You're in Toxic Overload! You may need to use several of the detox diets in this book to cleanse your system of toxins and develop new eating and lifestyle habits to prevent toxic overload in the future.

What Your Answers May Be Telling You

Although this short quiz is just the beginning of your detox journey, it may help you pinpoint some of the more obvious health issues affecting you. Here's a quick look at what some of your answers may be telling you, and how and why some of the detox diets in this book can help you accomplish your detox goals.

If you answered "yes" to questions 1 and 9, you may be consuming or retaining too much sodium (salt) as a result of diet, medications, lifestyle habits, or a combination of all three. Excess sodium causes bloating, water weight gain, and hypertension, or high blood pressure. Fortunately, several diets in this book can help you shed excess water in a healthy, delicious way, including the 5-Day Water Retention Flush, which focuses on low-sodium foods that help eliminate excess water, and the 15-Day Carb Flush, which acts as a natural diuretic. Both the 10-Day Raw Foods Detox and the 15-Day Vegan Detox will also help you reduce your sodium intake because they revolve around fresh fruits, vegetables, and whole grains that are naturally low in sodium.

If you answered "yes" to questions 4, 5, and 10, you may be a workaholic and/or city dweller who is regularly exposed to a wide variety of environmental toxins, including heavy metals, toxic fumes, cigarette smoke (yours and/or others), pesticides, toxic cleaning supplies, and excessive radiation from overhead wires, X-rays, and excessive use of computers and cell phones. The 30-Day Heavy Metal Detox revolves around nutrients that displace or bond to heavy metals in your body and neutralize their harmful effects.

If you answered "yes" to question 5 or 7, you may be overusing stimulants like caffeine and alcohol to keep you alert or relaxed, both of which may, in turn, be sabotaging your ability to get a good night's sleep. The 3-Day Juice Detox, the 10-Day Raw Foods Detox, and the 15-Day Vegan Detox, are loaded with antioxidants that will help calm and balance your body. If you've been consuming too much alcohol, the 7-Day Liver Detox will nourish your liver and help prevent serious diseases. (Note: This is not an alcohol detox diet.)

If you answered "yes" to questions 2 and 9, you're probably overweight or obese. Many of the detox diets in this book are low in carbohydrates, fats, cholesterol, and calories. By helping you shed pounds quickly and safely, they will also help reduce your risk of heart attack, stroke, diabetes, cancer, and other serious conditions. The diets include the 15-Day Mediterranean Detox, the 10-Day Cholesterol Flush, the 15-Day Carb Flush, the 10-Day Raw Foods Detox, and the 15-Day Vegan Detox.

If you answered "yes" to question 8, you may be allergic to lactose or gluten. This book contains the latest research on gluten and lactose intolerance, a 10-Day Lactose Detox and 10-Day Gluten Detox, and delicious recipes that are either lactose free or gluten free.

How to Use This Book

Once you've taken the quiz, decide which plan is best for you, and you're on your way! Each chapter explains the benefits of the detox diet and points you to the best foods to achieve your goal. You'll find meal plans and recipes that go along with each detox regimen. Note that some of the recommendations in the meal plans include recipes, while others do not. If the meal recommendation is not obvious and has no recipe associated with it, you'll find very simple tips for creating the dish following the entry. If you aren't familiar with the meal recommendations, a simple online search should turn up a recipe. Just remember to modify according to the detox guidelines. Most of the ingredients should be easy to find! However, if they aren't available at your local grocery store, you may need to seek out a specialty foods store—you'll be surprised by the number you'll find online.

Finally, always try to use fresh, organic fruits, vegetables, and meat whenever possible. Some packaged, store-bought ingredients will work, but make sure to read the ingredients list on the package so you know exactly what you're putting into your body and whether it is appropriate for your detox diet.

> **Food for Thought**
>
> *If you have diabetes or other blood sugar–related conditions, consult with your physician before embarking on any kind of detox diet, especially those that include fruit juice. In addition, if you are pregnant, nursing, or taking medication, you'll want to check with your doctor before starting a detox regimen.*

PART I

Fruit and Vegetable Detox Diets

Fruit and vegetable fasts and diets are the most popular type of detox diets. Ideal for total-body cleansing, losing weight, strengthening your immune system, and boosting energy, they contain fresh fruits and vegetables, or juices made from fresh fruits and vegetables. The four detox diets in this chapter include the 3-Day Juice Detox, the 15-Day Vegan Detox, the 10-Day Raw Foods Detox, and the 15-Day Mediterranean Detox. All four are rich in disease-fighting antioxidants and phytochemicals, vitamins, minerals, and electrolytes, and are very low in calories, sodium, saturated fat, and cholesterol. Although each detox diet has a slightly different purpose, you can mix and match the recipes in these four diets for endless variety.

Chapter 1

3-Day Juice Detox

A SHORT JUICE DETOX CAN BOOST YOUR IMMUNE SYSTEM, eliminate bloating, relieve constipation, and detox your total system. Fresh juices contain many vitamins, minerals, and antioxidants that cleanse the immune system and rid the body of free radicals and toxins that can set the stage for serious diseases. A 3-day detox is long enough to help cleanse your body, but not so long that it could lead to nutritional deficiencies.

Anatomy of a Juice Detox

If you've been eating a diet high in saturated fats, sugar, and salt, and low in fiber and nutrients, a short juice detox could be the health equivalent of spring-cleaning your body and giving it a healthy dose of disease-fighting antioxidants and fiber. Both are found in abundance in fresh fruits and vegetables.

Juice detoxing can give the body a much-needed "time out" from the "strenuous" work of digestion, and helps the immune system clear out dead, diseased, and damaged cells. Because juice contains little fiber, the amount of stool and frequency of elimination may be greatly reduced as the fast progresses.

A 3-day detox can be especially effective for breaking binges, cravings, and other bad eating habits.

> **Food for Thought**
> *If you're taking prescription drugs, consult with your pharmacist before including grapefruit or grapefruit juice in your diet because a compound in the fruit can alter the way they are metabolized and reduce or increase their effects in the body.*

The Best Way to Juice Detox

If you decide to go on a short juice detox, drink as much juice as you want and be sure to drink juices from a wide assortment of fruits and vegetables to ensure you consume a variety of vitamins, minerals, and antioxidants.

To strengthen your immune system, create juices from fruits and vegetables that contain natural healing properties, including beets, cabbage, wheatgrass, sprouts, lemon, carrots, celery, green peppers, oranges, parsley, apples, and grapefruit.

To shed excess water weight and eliminate bloating, consume produce that acts as a natural diuretic, including watermelon, parsley, cucumber, lemon, kiwi fruit, asparagus, and cantaloupe with the seed.

To relieve constipation or lose weight, mix bulking agents like psyllium husks and flax-seed in your homemade juices to promote regularity and keep you feeling full longer.

Four Steps to Get Started

You get more benefits from juice detoxing if you prepare your body for the challenge. For best results, follow these steps.

1. To begin the transition from solid to liquid foods, wean yourself off grains, breads, dairy, fish, and meat about 5 days before your fast, and consume a diet high in cooked vegetables, salads, fruits, and juices.
2. Start skipping a meal or two a couple of days prior to prepare your body for fasting.
3. The day before your fast, eat nothing but grapes, which have a strong detoxifying agent. Or consume only melons, apples, or citrus, which also have cleansing effects.
4. If you're new to fasting, consider doing a medically supervised fast at a health spa or clinic.

What to Expect

During a short detox lasting up to 3 days, your body changes the pH balance of your stomach, making it more alkaline. As your stomach contracts and your digestive tract is cleansed, you excrete large amounts of water, minerals, and water-soluble vitamins. As a result, you may experience hunger, headaches, light-headedness, copious urination, and weight loss.

How to Break a Fast

Although you may be tempted to eat everything in sight after coming off a juice detox, it's important to ease into normal eating to avoid stomach upset and stress to the system. Remember that while you were fasting, your stomach was essentially asleep. To "wake up" your digestive system without experiencing digestive distress, sit down when you eat, consume very small meals, eat slowly, and chew your food thoroughly.

> **DETOX TIP**
>
> Don't try to return too quickly to normal activity levels or exercise regimes. If you feel tired, rest.

Juicing Methods

There are different ways to juice and types of machines to use. Machines for juicing fruits and vegetables include the less expensive centrifugal juicer and the more expensive single- and twin-gear juicers, all of which extract the juice and run it through a fine sieve to separate it from the pulp. There are also ream-style juicers for citrus fruits. In the absence of a juicer, some opt to blend the fruits and veggies in a high-speed blender (like a Vitamix) and then strain the juice through a fine mesh bag. Juicers are so efficient at separating out the pulp, you don't need to worry about peeling vegetables or removing seeds from your fruit unless they are large pits. The seeds actually have nutritional value! Many people also juice the watermelon rind along with the flesh of the watermelon for the same reasons. Make sure to rinse or clean your produce well to remove dirt, small rocks, and unfriendly bacteria.

> **Food for Thought**
>
> *Although you may be tempted to do so, carrying out a juice detox for more than three days can have the potential for serious health consequences, including vitamin deficiencies, electrolyte imbalances, and more. You may feel "lighter" and more energetic after the detox, but going for longer than three days will make you feel more lethargic and less focused as your body tries to save energy. If you experience any negative symptoms during your 3-day detox, discontinue the plan and consult with your physician right away. If you have diabetes, make sure you consult with your physician before starting any kind of fruit juice detox regimen.*

Meal Plans for 3-Day Juice Detox

These meal options should be made with fresh, uncooked, organic fruit and vegetables in a juicer—not with store-bought juices, which can contain excess sugar and additives. Stir in filtered water very sparingly when needed to adjust to the desired consistency.

Day 1

Breakfast
Watermelon Straight-Up (page 7)
Papaya-Strawberry Juice (page 7)

Lunch
Apple Beeter (page 8)
Zucchini Juice (page 9)

Dinner
Green Apple-Broccoli Juice (page 10)
Sweet Potato-Carrot Juice (page 10)

Day 2

Breakfast
Apple-Blackberry Juice (2 red apples; 2 pints black-berries; 1 lemon, peeled)
Peach-Pineapple Juice (1 cup fresh pineapple; 1 peach, pitted)

Lunch
Broccoli-Apple-Carrot Juice (4 broccoli spears and crowns; ¼ cup Italian pars-ley; 2 Macintosh apples, cored; ¼ cup lemon juice)
Pineapple-Tangerine Juice (1 cup pineapple, peeled; 1 tangerine, peeled)

Dinner
Super Gallbladder Helper (page 12)
Broccoli Cabbage Patch (1 cup broccoli; ¼ small head red cabbage; 3 romaine lettuce leaves)

Day 3

Breakfast
Carrot-Parsley Juice (4 car-rots, peeled; ¼ cup Italian parsley; ¼ lemon, peeled)
Banana Cashew Smoothie (combine 1 banana and ½ cup cashews in a blender)

Lunch
Cherry-Cucumber Juice (1 cucumber, peeled; 2 cups cherries, pitted; 2 celery stalks, leaves intact)
Sweet Potato-Apple Juice (page 12)

Dinner
Salad in a Glass (1 cup broccoli; 3 butter lettuce leaves; 1 carrot; 2 red rad-ishes; 1 green onion)
Kokomo Coconut (1 papaya, seeded; ½ lime, peeled; 1 cup unsweetened coco-nut milk)
Watermelon-Lime-Cherry Juice (1 cup watermelon, rind removed; 1 cup cher-ries, pitted; ½ lime, peeled)

Recipes for 3-Day Juice Detox

Watermelon Straight-Up

Yield: 1 cup

INGREDIENTS

1 cup watermelon chunks

1 lime, peeled

Juice watermelon and lime. Stir.

80 calories | .75 g fat, .01 g saturated fat | 16.98 g carbohydrate | 1.26 g protein | 4 mg sodium | .72 g fiber

What Is Papain?

Papayas contain papain, a digestive enzyme that aids in the breakdown of protein. Papaya is a very good source of vitamins A and C.

Papaya Strawberry Juice

Yield: 1¼ cups

INGREDIENTS

2 papayas, cut into chunks

1 cup strawberries, no need to hull

Juice papayas and strawberries. Stir.

295 calories | 1.2 g fat, .28 g saturated fat | 66.66 g carbohydrate | 4.32 g protein | 19 mg sodium | 7.98 g fiber

What's So Great about Blueberries?

Low in calories (½ cup has just 40 calories) and high in antioxidants, these sweet yet tart fruits pack a nutritious punch. Blueberries also help enhance memory and lower cholesterol.

Recipes for 3-Day Juice Detox

Blueberry-Banana Juice

Yield: 1½ cups

INGREDIENTS
2 cups blueberries
1 banana, peeled

Juice blueberries. Blend blueberry juice and banana in blender. Stir.

227 calories | 1.24 g fat, .19 g saturated fat | 51.69 g carbohydrate | 2.37 g protein | 13 mg sodium | 10.1 g fiber

Apple Beeter

Yield: 1 cup

INGREDIENTS
1 beet
2 red apples

Juice apples and beet. Stir.

307 calories | 1.58 g fat, .26 g saturated fat | 71 g carbohydrate | 2.24 g protein | 72 g sodium | 8.8 g fiber

Is There a Bitter Taste to Your Juice?
If any of your juices are too bitter for your taste, apples are a perfect sweetener.

Recipes for 3-Day Juice Detox

Zucchini Juice

Yield: 1½ cups

INGREDIENTS
1 green zucchini
3 carrots
2 red apples

Juice zucchini, carrots, and apples. Stir.

193 calories | 1 g fat, .17 g saturated fat | 43.64 g carbohydrate | 2.36 g protein | 40 mg sodium | 5.46 g fiber

Carrot-Cucumber-Beet Juice

Yield: 1¼ cups

INGREDIENTS
3 carrots
1 cucumber
1 beet

Juice carrots, cucumber, and beet. Stir.

126 calories | .63 g fat, 1.2 g saturated fat | 26.88 g carbohydrate | 3.15 g protein | 79 mg sodium | 3.27 g fiber

What Color Are Beets?

Beets come in many colors from deep red to orange. Beets can also be white. The Chioggia is called a candy cane beet and has rings of white and red. Small or medium beets are more tender than larger ones.

Recipes for 3-Day Juice Detox

Green Apple-Broccoli Juice

Yield: 1½ cups

INGREDIENTS
2 Granny Smith apples
1 orange, peeled
⅛ cup Italian parsley
1 cup broccoli

Juice apples and orange. Juice broccoli and Italian parsley. Stir.

---

173 calories | .95 g fat, .15 g saturated fat | 38.94 g carbohydrate | 2.25 g protein | 13 mg sodium | 10.88 g fiber

Why Choose Italian (Flat-Leaf) Parsley?

Italian parsley is packed with chlorophyll, vitamins A and C, calcium, magnesium, phosphorous, potassium, sodium, and sulfur. It helps stimulate oxygen metabolism, cell respiration, and regeneration. Choose parsley with no signs of wilting and bright green leaves.

Sweet Potato-Carrot Juice

Yield: 1 cup

INGREDIENTS
2 carrots
1 medium sweet potato

Juice carrots and sweet potato. Stir.

---

237 calories | .75 g fat, .15 g saturated fat | 53.47 g carbohydrate | 4.13 g protein | 71 mg sodium | 2.86 g fiber

What Is Colitis?

Colitis means that the colon is inflamed. Colitis is associated with irritable bowel syndrome and it includes attacks of diarrhea, stomach cramps, and sometimes constipation. It can be brought on by stress, poor diet, and/or food allergies. Carrots and sweet potatoes are among the foods that help with colon problems.

Recipes for 3-Day Juice Detox

Super Melon Juice

Yield: 1½ cups

INGREDIENTS

1 cup watermelon chunks

1 cup cantaloupe chunks

1 orange, peeled

Juice melons and orange. Stir.

86 calories | .63 g fat, .01 g saturated fat | 18.31 g carbohydrate | 1.67 g protein | 9 mg sodium | 2.08 g fiber

What Makes This So "Super"?

This recipe provides fruits that are rich in beta-carotene, vitamin C, and potassium.

Orange-Beet Juice

Yield: ¾ cup

INGREDIENTS

2 oranges, peeled

1 beet

Juice beet and oranges. Stir.

151 calories | .38 g fat, .05 g saturated fat | 33.5 g carbohydrate | 3.36 g protein | 72 mg sodium | 7 g fiber

Why Are Beets the Best?

Beets are superfoods that help cleanse the liver and gallbladder, detox the lymphatic system, and even reverse and/or prevent cancers induced by radiation—and that's just for starters. The beets, greens, and roots are all highly nutritious and packed with calcium, potassium, and vitamins A and C.

Recipes for 3-Day Juice Detox

Super Gallbladder Helper

Yield: 4 cups

INGREDIENTS

1 bunch spinach, rinsed well

1 cucumber

½ bunch celery, with leaves

1 bunch Italian parsley

½-inch piece fresh gingerroot

2 apples

½ lime, peeled

Juice ingredients in order listed. Stir.

99 calories | .7 g fat, .12 g saturated fat | 20.49 g carbohydrate | 2.59 g protein | 58 mg sodium | 2.97 g fiber

What Does a Green Juice Do for Me?

Green juice provides a great deal of chlorophyll, which some believe increases the flow of oxygen in our bodies. Dark green leafy vegetables can help with gallbladder problems

Sweet Potato-Apple Juice

Yield: 1 cup

INGREDIENTS

1 sweet potato

2 Granny Smith apples

Juice sweet potato and apples. Stir.

230 calories | 1.92 g fat, .34 g saturated fat | 99.85 g carbohydrate | 3.4 g protein | 21 mg sodium | 18.96 g fiber

What's in an Apple?

Rich in vitamins A, B1, B2, B6, and C; folic acid; biotin; and a host of minerals that promote healthy skin, hair, and nails, apples also contain pectin, a fiber that absorbs toxins, stimulates digestion, and helps reduce cholesterol. Apples are extremely versatile, and blend well with other juices.

Chapter 2

15-Day Vegan Detox

WHAT DO WOODY HARRELSON, ALICIA SILVERSTONE, JOAQUIN PHOENIX, Natalie Portman, Pamela Anderson, and Paul McCartney have in common? They are all vegans or ultrastrict vegetarians who don't consume beef, poultry, fish, seafood, or animal by-products such as eggs, dairy, and honey. Adopting a vegan diet can help prevent heart disease, diabetes, and lower blood pressure.

The Skinny on Vegan Diets

Vegan diets supply all the nutrients you need in a delicious way that eliminates dangerous fats and cholesterol.

Unlike the Standard American Diet (SAD), which revolves around animal-based protein, vegan diets revolve around protein-rich plant products. These include soy (tempeh and tofu), which has no saturated fat or cholesterol; and wheat gluten, a high-protein food often called the "wheat meat," which has a chewy texture and is used in vegan meatloaf, barbecue "ribs," and other faux meat dishes. Other good sources of plant protein include lentils, chickpeas, peanut butter, almonds, spinach, rice, whole wheat bread, potatoes, kale, and broccoli.

Studies show the average American eats twice as much protein as is needed and far too much saturated fat, processed foods, and sugar. By going on a vegan diet, you can reduce your intake of all these foods and lower your risk of heart attack, stroke, and obesity. A balanced vegan diet containing a variety of fruits, vegetables, nuts, seeds, grains, and legumes will provide plenty of protein. With meat at the center of the plate, the SAD has promoted the notion that we need more protein than is necessary.

Vegans can also easily fulfill their daily calcium needs by consuming products fortified with calcium, including soy milk, orange juice, and tofu. Many fruits and vegetables are also naturally high in calcium, including almonds, brown rice, oranges, broccoli, kale, collard greens, parsley, beet greens, watercress, spinach, romaine lettuce, and string beans.

A vegan diet also provides excellent levels of zinc, which repairs tissue and reduces inflammation. Great sources include pumpkin seeds, peanuts, peanut butter, and fortified cereals. Gingerroot, parsley, turnips, carrots, grapes, spinach, lettuce, cabbage, tangerines, and cucumbers also supply zinc.

Plant foods are also rich in nonheme iron, a type of iron that helps build red blood cells. Nonheme iron is found in dried fruits like raisins, dates, prunes, and apricots, as well as parsley, broccoli, cauliflower, asparagus, strawberries, chard, blackberries, cabbage, beets with greens, carrots, and pineapple.

DETOX TIP

You don't have to wear a milk mustache to fulfill your daily calcium requirements. Just 1 cup of raw sesame seeds or tofu supplies more calcium than 1 cup of low-fat milk. In addition to building strong bones and teeth, calcium also helps regulate normal blood pressure.

Food for Thought

The body has an easier time absorbing heme iron, the kind found in animal products, than nonheme iron, the kind found in plants. If you're on a vegan diet, consider boosting your body's absorption of iron by eating more vitamin C–rich foods, including citrus fruit, peppers, dark leafy greens, asparagus, cabbage, strawberries, broccoli, and cauliflower.

10 Reasons to Go Vegan

According to research in *Vegetarian Journal*, people who consumed a vegan diet for at least three years had lower blood pressure, lower blood triglyceride levels, and lower fasting blood glucose levels than nonvegans. Based on the study, researchers concluded that vegans were at a lower risk of developing heart disease and type-2 diabetes than nonvegans. Here are ten reasons why you should go vegan.

1. Vegan diets are high in fiber, which promotes regularity and helps fight colon cancer.
2. Vegan diets are rich in potassium, which balances water and acidity in your body, and stimulates the kidneys to eliminate toxins. Studies show that diets high in potassium also reduce the risk of cardiovascular diseases and cancer.

3. Vegan diets are naturally high in phytochemicals—substances found in plants that fight free radicals and help protect the body from premature aging and cancer.

4. Vegan diets are high in vitamin E, which builds a healthy heart and protects your skin, eyes, and brain from free radical damage. Vitamin E is found in dark leafy greens, nuts, and whole grains.

5. Studies show that consuming a vegan diet high in fresh fruits and vegetables can greatly reduce the risk of prostate, colon, and breast cancer. Women living in countries where very little meat and animal products are consumed have lower rates of breast cancer than women living in countries where diets revolve around animal products.

6. Vegan diets may help you lose weight by eliminating many foods that cause weight gain, including cholesterol and saturated fat. According to research, vegans have a lower Body Mass Index (BMI) than nonvegans—which is an indicator of a healthy weight.

7. Studies show that vegetarians live three to six years longer than nonvegetarians.

8. By eliminating dairy and red meat from their diets, vegans report a dramatic reduction in body odor and bad breath, according to studies.

9. Research indicates that women who switch to vegan diets have fewer or less intense PMS symptoms because they no longer consume dairy products. However, there are physicians on both sides of this issue—those who say dairy causes PMS, and those who say it reduces PMS symptoms. The idea that dairy causes PMS is based on the rise in blood estrogen levels due to the saturated fat these products often contain. In contrast, PMS symptom reduction seems to be a function of improved calcium levels.

10. Studies show that eliminating dairy, meat, and eggs may help reduce the incidence of migraine headaches and such allergic symptoms as nasal congestion.

Those Amazing Antioxidants and Mighty Phytochemicals

Vegan diets are high in antioxidants, the heroes of the nutrition world. Antioxidants are substances that protect your cells against the effects of free radicals. Free radicals are molecules produced when your body breaks down food or when you're exposed to environmental toxins such as tobacco smoke, radiation, and pollution. In addition, free radicals may damage cells and may play a role in the development of heart disease, cancer, and many other diseases.

Fruits and vegetables are also high in phytochemicals—nonnutritive plant chemicals with protective or disease preventive properties. There are more than 1,000 known phytochemicals, although scientists believe there are thousands more yet to be discovered. Although fruits and vegetables produce phytochemicals to protect themselves from illness and attack, research shows these chemicals also protect humans from diseases.

Most phytochemicals protect cells against oxidative damage and reduce the risk of developing certain types of cancer. Some of the more well-known phytochemicals include:

- lycopene (found in tomatoes)
- isoflavones (found in soy)
- flavonoids (found in fruits)
- saponins (found in beans)
- capsaicin (found in hot peppers)
- allyl sulfides (found in onions, leeks, and garlic)
- carotenoids (found in fruits and carrots)
- polyphenols (found in tea and grapes)
- indoles (found in cruciferous veggies)

Other Great Stuff in Fruits and Veggies

In addition to antioxidants and phytochemicals, produce is packed with the following nutrients that are essential for health.

Amino Acids: The building blocks of protein, amino acids comprise more than half of your body's nonwater weight.

Carbohydrates: Fruits are high in both simple and complex carbohydrates. These quickly absorbed molecules provide a ready source of energy. Complex carbohydrates, found in root vegetables and potatoes, are broken down more slowly than simple carbohydrates found in sweeter fruits like apples, oranges, and cherries. By releasing a more gradual supply of sugar, complex carbs help maintain steady glucose levels, which is especially important for diabetics.

Chlorophyll: Chlorophyll helps your body's organs (especially your liver) eliminate toxins by improving cellular and organ detoxification. Chlorophyll can also prevent carcinogens from binding to the DNA in your body's cells. In addition, chlorophyll helps the body maintain a proper acid-alkaline balance. This is especially important today because most Americans eat a diet that is extremely high in acids and low in alkaline foods. Studies show that a high-acid environment in the body may predispose it to cancer.

Chlorophyll also protects against the formation of calcium stones in the kidney.

Essential amino acids: These eight amino acids are responsible for thousands of bodily functions, including repairing and building muscle, blood, and organs; manufacturing hormones; maintaining a healthy immune system; mental functions; circulation; sleep; memory; and physical and mental energy. Because they are not manufactured by the body, they must be supplied from the food you eat.

Enzymes: These biochemicals act as catalysts to trigger a wide variety of functions in your body, including regenerating and maintaining fluids, cells, tissues, and organs. Researchers have identified about 1,000 enzymes, many of which are found in fresh fruits and vegetables. Without enzymes, your body can't carry out necessary functions or make the most of nutrients found in other foods.

Fats: While fat is often vilified, your body needs a small amount of healthy unsaturated fat for bodily functions. Good sources include avocados, olives, nuts, and seeds, as well as heart-healthy oils and butters derived from olives, almonds, walnuts, and safflower and sunflower seeds.

Fiber: Fiber is type of carbohydrate found in fruits and vegetables that resists your body's efforts to digest it via enzymes and acids. Soluble fiber forms a gel-like substance in your digestive tract that binds cholesterol so it can't be reabsorbed. Insoluble fiber, which is often called "nature's broom," decreases the time food spends in your intestine before it is eliminated as waste. Many fruits and vegetables are loaded with fiber.

> **DETOX TIP**
>
> It is essential to stay hydrated during any detox diet. Drink at least eight glasses of filtered water a day. Or choose fresh juices to replenish lost fluids while also providing vitamins, minerals, enzymes, and phytochemicals.

Minerals: Minerals are found in abundance in fresh fruits and vegetables, and especially in organic produce. Minerals like calcium and magnesium are important for building and repairing bones, teeth, hair, and nails; while potassium, sodium, chloride, and calcium are essential for regulating the body's balance of electrolytes. Trace minerals, or minerals needed by the body in minuscule amounts, including chromium, copper, fluoride, boron, and selenium, play an important role in many bodily functions, including metabolism and the growth of hair and nails.

Vitamins are substances necessary to sustain life. Fruits and vegetables provide a wide array of essential vitamins, including carotenes, vitamin A, vitamin B2 (riboflavin), vitamin B3 (niacin), vitamin B5 (pantothenic acid), vitamin B6 (pyridoxine), vitamin B7 (biotin), vitamin B9 (folic acid), and vitamins C, E, and K.

Lifestyle Benefits

In addition to the health benefits above, by following a vegan lifestyle, you'll be helping the environment and global food supply. Growing plants for food takes far less resources than growing animals for food. By consuming organic produce, you'll also avoid consuming dangerous pesticides and herbicides.

By avoiding animal products, you'll also reduce your exposure to bacteria like *E. coli* and salmonella, both caused by eating contaminated animal products, and avoid contracting a fatal condition like mad cow disease. Many farm animals are fed high amounts of antibiotics and hormones. By eliminating meat from your diet, you may reduce your risk of developing bacterial resistance to antibiotics and of ingesting excess hormones, which can disrupt your normal hormone balance and lead to the growth of tumors.

> **Food for Thought**
> *Following a vegan diet may inhibit healthy digestion by eliminating essential acids and enzymes found in animal protein that are necessary for digestion. In addition, because vegans are at risk for deficiencies of vitamin B12, iron, calcium, omega-3 fatty acids and possibly vitamin D, it is important to take care to include foods fortified with these nutrients or take supplements to prevent these deficiencies. If you decide to adopt a vegan diet beyond this 15-day plan, you may want to seek the advice of a nutritionist.*

Meal Plans for 15-Day Vegan Detox

The idea with this vegan detox plan is to eliminate all dairy, eggs, and meat from your diet for a few weeks. There are several milk substitutes on the market, so feel free to experiment with soymilk, nut milks, and even coconut milk! For Days 8–15, go to Day 1 and repeat the sequence.

Day 1

Breakfast

1 serving Tofu Scramble (page 22)
1 slice Whole Wheat Toast with Fresh Preserves
Herbal Tea or Coffee

Lunch

1 cup Roasted Tomato and Red Bell Pepper Soup (page 23)
½ cup Easy Vegetarian Chili with Brown Rice, Kidney Beans, Corn, Tomatoes, and Chili Powder
Herbal Tea

Dinner

½ cup Broccoli Corn Tomato Sauté (page 24)
1 Pita Pocket with Garbanzo Beans, Chopped Veggies, and Italian Dressing
2-inch square Double-Chocolate Brownie (page 25)
Herbal Tea

Day 2

Breakfast

2 Apple-Cinnamon Waffles (made with soymilk) with Maple Syrup
1 cup Sliced Cantaloupe
Herbal Tea or Coffee

Lunch

1 Grilled Soy Cheese Sandwich on Whole Wheat Bread
1 cup Vegetarian Vegetable Soup
Herbal Tea

Dinner

1 serving Tomatoes Stuffed with Black Bean Salad (page 26)
1 cup Garden Salad
1 cup Fruit Salad (with watermelon, pineapple, and blueberries)
Herbal Tea

Day 3

Breakfast

6 ounces Orange Juice
1 cup Soy Yogurt with Berries
1 slice Whole Wheat Toast with Nut Butter
Herbal Tea

Lunch

Sautéed Spinach and White Beans with 1 cup Grilled Polenta (made with vegan margarine, like Earth Balance brand)
1 cup Butter Lettuce Salad with Dried Cherries and Pine Nuts (page 27)
½ Grapefruit Sections with Fresh Strawberries
Herbal Tea

Dinner

1 cup Curried Vegetable Stew (page 28)
1 cup Spinach Salad with Tahini Dressing
1 Grilled Pear with a Drizzle of Agave Syrup and Cinnamon
Herbal Tea

Day 4

Breakfast

Fresh Grapefruit Juice
1 cup Oatmeal with Apples, Walnuts, and Raisins
Herbal Tea

Lunch

1 Vegan Burger with Soy Cheese on a Whole Wheat Bun, with Lettuce, Tomato, and Onion
¾ cup Vegan Summer Potato Salad (page 29)
1 cup Fresh-Squeezed Lemonade with Sliced Fresh Strawberries

Dinner

1 cup Tuscan-Style Penne (page 30)
1 cup Leafy Green Salad with Olive Oil Dressing
¾ cup Rainbow Sorbet
Herbal Tea

Day 5

Breakfast

1 serving Tofu Scramble (page 22)
8 ounces Cranberry Juice with Seltzer Water
Herbal Tea

Lunch

1 cup Spinach Salad with Oranges, Sesame Seeds, and Sesame Dressing
1 slice Whole Wheat Bread with Fresh Preserves and Nut Butter
Herbal Tea

Dinner

4 ounces Lentil Loaf (page 31)
½ cup Mashed Potatoes with Chives (made with soymilk and vegan margarine)
1 cup Leafy Green Salad with Pesto Dressing
¾ cup Chocolate Soy Pudding with a Sliced Banana
Herbal Tea

Day 6

Breakfast

1 sliced Vegan Sausage and Soy Cheese on Whole Wheat Toast
6 ounces Orange Juice
Herbal Tea

Lunch

1½ cups Spaghetti Marinara with Mushrooms and Olives
1 slice Toasted Italian Bread (rubbed with fresh garlic and drizzled with olive oil)
1 cup Fresh Garden Salad
Herbal Tea

Dinner

1½ cups Rice Vegetable Casserole (page 32)
1 cup Chopped Zucchini Salad
1 slice Tofu Cheesecake with Berries
Herbal Tea

Meal Plans for 15-Day Vegan Detox

Breakfast

1 Banana Muffin (use applesauce, soymilk, or oil as a binder instead of eggs or milk)
1 cup Fresh Fruit with Soy Yogurt
Herbal Tea

Lunch

1 cup Vegetarian Chili
1 ounce Tortilla Chips
½ Avocado Stuffed with Chopped Veggies
1 Vegan Chocolate Chip Cookie
Herbal Tea

Dinner

1½ cups Pasta with Portobello Mushrooms (sautéed in olive oil with 2 minced garlic cloves)
1 cup Garden Salad with Olive Oil Dressing
Herbal Tea
1 slice Date Nut Bread (using vegan margarine and mashed banana as a binder)

Tofu Scramble

Serves: 2

INGREDIENTS

6 ounces firm tofu, drained

½ white onion, diced small

½ red bell pepper, diced

2 tablespoons extra-virgin olive oil

1 teaspoon garlic powder

salt and pepper to taste

1 teaspoon Italian parsley, minced

½ cup salsa

Slice tofu into cubes.

Sauté onion, bell pepper, and tofu in olive oil over low heat.

Stir constantly.

Add garlic powder, salt, and pepper.

Serve with salsa and minced parsley.

251 calories | 19.1 g fat | 11.52 g carbohydrate | 8.17 g protein | 244 mg sodium | .6 g fiber

What's Up with Soy?

Unlike the SAD, which revolves around animal-based protein, vegan diets revolve around protein-rich plant products, including soy (tempeh and tofu), which are great sources of protein containing less fat, cholesterol, and sodium than their meat counterparts.

Recipes for 15-Day Vegan Detox

Roasted Tomato and Red Bell Pepper Soup

Serves: 3

INGREDIENTS

2 pounds Roma tomatoes, cut in half

1 medium onion, thinly sliced

2 large red bell peppers, seeded and quartered

3 large garlic heads, top cut off

2 tablespoons extra-virgin olive oil

Kosher salt and fresh cracked

black pepper to taste

2 cups vegetable broth

1 teaspoon fresh thyme

What's the Perfect Quartet for Fighting Disease?

Tomatoes, peppers, onions, and garlic are all loaded with antioxidants, which help fight free radicals that damage cells and cause disease and premature aging.

Heat oven to 400°F. Place tomatoes, onion, and peppers on large baking sheet. Add garlic and coat everything with a light drizzle of extra-virgin olive oil. Add kosher salt and pepper.

Place in oven and roast for 35–45 minutes or until vegetables are brown and soft. Cool. Peel garlic gloves.

Place vegetables and peeled garlic cloves in blender with vegetable broth. Blend until smooth.

Add thyme and adjust seasoning.

Chill soup until very cold.

---

285 calories | 12 g fat | 38 g carbohydrate | 6 g protein | 649 mg sodium | 3.5 g fiber

Recipes for 15-Day Vegan Detox

Broccoli Corn Tomato Sauté

Serves: 2

INGREDIENTS

1½ cups broccoli, cut into florets

1 tablespoon extra-virgin olive oil

¾ cup frozen corn

2 small Roma tomatoes, diced

½ teaspoon garlic, minced

1 tablespoon dried marjoram

1 tablespoon vegetable broth

Kosher salt and black pepper to taste

Sauté broccoli in olive oil. Add corn, tomatoes, garlic, and marjoram.

Add vegetable broth and cover pan with lid.

Steam until broccoli is crisp tender and corn is warmed through.

Add salt and pepper to taste.

232 calories | 13 g fat | 23 g carbohydrate | 5 g protein | 140 mg sodium | 2 g fiber

Why Is Broccoli So Great for Vegans?

Packed with fiber to promote regularity, broccoli is surprisingly high in plant protein, which makes it a great choice for vegans. Sulforaphane, a phytochemical found in cruciferous vegetables, helps stimulate enzymes in the body that detoxify carcinogens before they have a chance to damage cells.

Double Chocolate Brownies

Serves: 8

INGREDIENTS

1½ cups whole wheat flour

1 cup unsweetened cocoa powder

¼ teaspoon sea salt

10 ounces soft silken tofu

1 teaspoon pure vanilla extract

1 teaspoon orange extract

½ cup barley malt

½ cup maple syrup

1 cup low-fat soy or rice milk

⅔ cup chopped walnuts

Combine flour, cocoa, and salt in medium bowl.

In blender, puree tofu, orange and vanilla extracts, barley malt, maple syrup, and milk.

Stir tofu mixture into flour mixture, add nuts and mix well.

Pour into lightly oiled 8" × 8" baking dish and bake at 350°F for 30 minutes.

Cut into eight 2" × 4" pieces.

320 calories | 10 g fat | 54 g carbohydrate | 9 g protein | 148 mg sodium | 6 g. fiber

What's Another Reason to Love Chocolate?

Dark chocolate is a superfood that's loaded with disease-fighting antioxidants as well as epicatechin, a compound that promotes functional changes in a part of the brain involved with learning and memory.

Recipes for 15-Day Vegan Detox

Black Bean Salad

Serves: 4

INGREDIENTS

2 teaspoons Dijon mustard

⅛ cup fresh lime juice

1 teaspoon lime zest

2 tablespoons apple cider vinegar

1 tablespoon sugar

1 teaspoon cumin

1 teaspoon garlic powder

½ tablespoon extra-virgin olive oil

Salt and black pepper, to taste

2 ears corn on the cob, steamed and kernels removed

15-ounce can black beans, rinsed and drained

¼ cup green onion, washed and sliced

1 tablespoon fresh cilantro, minced

To make dressing, whisk Dijon mustard, lime juice, zest, vinegar and sugar. Add cumin and garlic. Whisk in olive oil and taste for flavor. Add salt and pepper as needed.

Mix corn, black beans, green onion, and cilantro together.

Toss with vinaigrette.

This salad will keep for several days in the refrigerator.

---

415 calories | 26 g fat | 33 g carbohydrate | 10 g protein | 595 mg sodium | 2.4 g fiber

Do You Know Your Beans?

Packed with protein and fiber, beans are to vegetarians what meat is to carnivores. Beans also provide lots of disease-fighting phytochemicals, and bioactive compounds like isoflavones, which are believed to help protect against cancer.

Recipes for 15-Day Vegan Detox

Butter Lettuce Salad with Dried Cherries and Pine Nuts

Serves: 2

INGREDIENTS

1 head butter lettuce

¼ cup balsamic vinegar

1 tablespoon honey or agave syrup

1 teaspoon Dijon mustard

¼ cup extra-virgin olive oil

Salt and pepper, to taste

2 teaspoons pine nuts, toasted

⅛ cup dried cherries, halved

Is Butter Lettuce Really a Nutritional Zero?

Contrary to popular belief, butter lettuce is not a nutritional dud. One head of lettuce provides more than seven times the RDA for vitamin A, 3.5 times the RDA for vitamin C, and more than a third of the RDA for thiamine, iron, and potassium. A head of lettuce also supplies about 25 percent of your daily needs for calcium, vitamin B6, and magnesium, and a nice dose of phosphorous, copper, and zinc.

Tear lettuce into bite-size pieces and place in bowl.

Stir balsamic vinegar and honey into Dijon.

Drizzle olive oil in while whisking constantly.

Season dressing with salt and pepper to taste.

Toss dressing over lettuce leaves. Place in bowls and top with nuts and cherries.

---

322 calories | 29 g fat | 13 g carbohydrate | 2 g protein | 68 mg sodium | 1 g fiber

Recipes for 15-Day Vegan Detox

Curried Vegetable Stew

Serves: 2

INGREDIENTS

2 teaspoons extra-virgin olive oil

1 onion, diced into medium-size chunks

1 sweet potato, peeled and cut into medium-size chunks

1 zucchini, cut into 1-inch chunks

1 green bell pepper, cut into ¾-inch pieces

2 tablespoons curry powder

1 teaspoon cumin

1 tablespoon minced garlic

1 (15-ounce) can garbanzo beans, drained and rinsed

1 (14-ounce) can diced tomatoes and their juice

1 cup low-sodium vegetable broth

½ teaspoon each salt and pepper

Heat olive oil and sauté onion, sweet potato, zucchini, and green pepper.

Cook 10 minutes or until vegetables are golden brown.

Add curry and cumin and cook for an additional minute, stirring constantly. Add garlic and sauté for 30 seconds.

Add garbanzo beans, tomatoes and their juice, vegetable broth, salt, and pepper. Cook over high heat until mixture comes to a boil. Reduce heat to medium low and cover. Simmer for 10 minutes or until vegetables are tender.

365 calories | 11 g fat | 46 g carbohydrate | 20 g protein | 1,290 mg sodium | 5 g fiber

What's So Great about Zucchini?

Rich in vitamin B, niacin, calcium, and potassium, zucchini has a bland flavor that blends in well with many other vegetables. It also helps cleanse and soothe the bladder and kidneys.

Recipes for 15-Day Vegan Detox

Vegan Summer Potato Salad

Serves: 6

INGREDIENTS

2½ cups boiled red or white potatoes, cooled and cut into 1-inch cubes

⅛ cup diced onion

⅛ cup diced celery

⅛ cup zucchini, thinly sliced into half-moons

⅛ cup radishes, thinly sliced into half-moons

⅛ cup grated carrot

½ cup Vegenaise or other vegan mayonnaise

¼ teaspoon yellow mustard

½ teaspoon sweet pickle relish

1 tablespoons diced dill pickle

Salt and fresh cracked black pepper to taste

Combine potatoes, onion, celery, zucchini, radishes, and carrots in a medium bowl.

To make the dressing, mix the vegan mayonnaise, yellow mustard, sweet pickle relish, and dill pickles in a small bowl.

Pour dressing over potatoes and vegetables and mix carefully to avoid breaking up potatoes. Add salt and fresh cracked black pepper to taste. Chill for 1 hour.

181 calories | 12 g fat | 14 g carbohydrate | 1 g protein | 140 mg sodium | 1 g fiber

Can Vegans Have Their Mayo and Eat It Too?

While traditional mayonnaise is egg based and therefore not vegan friendly, Follow Your Heart's Vegenaise and other brands of vegan mayos are eggless and made with heart-healthy oils, such as canola and grape seed oil. Vegan mayonnaise can be found at health food stores, high-end super-markets, and many chain grocery stores.

Recipes for 15-Day Vegan Detox

Tuscan-Style Penne

Serves: 2

INGREDIENTS

4 ounces whole wheat penne pasta, uncooked

1 large garlic clove, crushed

1 tablespoon extra-virgin olive oil

1 cup baby spinach leaves

½ cup roasted red bell peppers

1 (15-ounce) can cannellini beans, drained and rinsed

1 tablespoon fresh basil, chopped

Salt and pepper to taste

4 tablespoons vegan Parmesan "cheese"

Cook pasta in boiling water. Drain.

Sauté garlic in olive oil. Add spinach and sauté until wilted.

Add roasted red peppers and beans.

Add pasta to sauté pan and mix in basil and salt and pepper.

Serve pasta topped with additional basil and vegan Parmesan.

---

358 calories | 10 g fat | 97 g carbohydrate | 29 g protein | 629 mg sodium | 7 g fiber

What's In Vegan Parmesan Cheese?

Any vegan Parmesan cheese will do, but try vegan Parmesan cheese made with ground-up walnuts and spices. High in omega-3 fatty acids and vitamin B12, it's a great nondairy topping for pasta, pizza, and steamed veggies. Look for it online or in health food stores or high-end supermarkets.

Lentil Loaf

Serves 4

INGREDIENTS

1 cups cooked lentils

1 cup quick oatmeal

½ cup onion, chopped

1 clove garlic, minced

2 cups tomato sauce

1½ teaspoon Italian herb seasoning

Preheat oven to 350°F.

Combine all ingredients and salt and pepper to taste in a bowl. Mix thoroughly and press mixture into a lightly oiled loaf pan.

Bake 50 minutes or until loaf is cooked through.

Love those Lentils

Lentils are an excellent source of protein, fiber, and folic acid. Because they are so high in fiber they said to aid in lowering cholesterol and managing diabetes.

235 calories | 1.9 g fat | 43.8 g carbohydrate | 13.8g protein | 745 mg sodium | 13.2 g fiber

Recipes for 15-Day Vegan Detox

Rice Vegetable Casserole

Serves: 6

INGREDIENTS

¾ cup brown rice, uncooked

1½ cups water

1 (15-ounce) can black beans, rinsed

1 (15-ounce) can no-salt corn, drained

1 (15-ounce) can diced tomatoes with green chilies

1 cup salsa

1 cup vegan sour cream

¼ teaspoon each salt and pepper

½ cup red onion, chopped

¼ cup pitted black olives, sliced

In a large saucepan, bring rice and water to boil. Reduce heat, cover and simmer for 40 minutes or until rice is cooked through.

In a large bowl, combine beans, rice, corn, tomatoes, salsa, sour cream, and salt and pepper.

Place rice mixture into an 8" × 8" glass dish coated lightly with oil.

Top with black olives and red onion

Bake covered with foil at 350°F for 30 minutes.

267 calories | 1.67 g fat | 52.3 g carbohydrate | 10.6 g protein | 628 mg sodium | 2.64 g fiber

Why Is Brown Rice Healthier Than White Rice?

White rice undergoes a refining process that destroys many of its nutrients and zaps 67 percent of its vitamin B3, 80 percent of its vitamin B1, 90 percent of its vitamin B6, 50 percent of its manganese and phosphorous, 60 percent of its iron, and 100 percent of its dietary fiber and essential fatty acids. White rice is then "enriched" to replace only a small percentage of what was lost through processing. That's why most vegans prefer to make brown rice a staple of their diet.

Chapter 3

10-Day Raw Foods Detox

RAW FOODS DIETS ARE QUICKLY BECOMING MORE POPULAR among health-conscious people. The raw foods diet provides most of the nutrients necessary for health and disease prevention and may help prevent everyday ailments like headaches and allergies. Followers of the raw food movement, also called "raw foodists," believe that cooking foods above 118°F releases harmful toxins and destroys 90 percent of the natural enzymes in fruits, vegetables, nuts, and grains.

The Details of a Raw Foods Diet

A raw foods diet revolves around 75–100 percent unprocessed and uncooked plant foods, including fruits and vegetables, nuts, seeds, sprouted beans and grains, and sea vegetables, with an emphasis on organic produce.

Other foods permitted on raw vegan diets may include vinegars and foods cured in vinegar, pure maple syrup, agave syrup, stevia, soy sauce, fermented foods like sauerkraut and miso, cold-pressed oils, raw nut butters, and raw nut "milks."

Even though some people see it as a concern, it's easy to consume enough protein on a raw foods diet, or 25 to 30 grams daily. Many plant-based foods, including nuts and legumes, are very high in protein and can also be eaten raw. The best liquids to drink on a raw foods diet are unprocessed beverages that are free of preservatives and additives. These include purified (not tap) water, homemade (not bottled) juices, coconut water or coconut milk made from a young coconut, and tea brewed by the sun. Soft drinks, bottled drinks, coffee, and alcohol are not permitted.

> **DETOX TIP**
>
> Not everything you eat on a raw foods diet must be raw or cold. You can heat foods up in a dehydrator, warming plate, or coffee maker to 118°F, the temperature at which heat begins to destroy nutrients.

The Benefits of a Raw Food Diet

Raw foodists claim raw or "living" foods contain enzymes that are destroyed by cooking, rendering food less nutritious and more toxic. They claim enzymes in raw foods not only help you digest and absorb the foods you eat, but also prevent toxicity that results in overweight and obesity.

A raw foods diet increases energy and skin tone, promotes weight loss and healthy digestion, and helps reduce heart disease because the diet has low levels of trans fats, saturated fats, and sodium, and high levels of fiber, disease-fighting antioxidants, and phytochemicals.

In addition, raw food diets exclude unhealthy foods that have been processed, canned, bottled, prepackaged, or "adulterated" through the addition of preservatives, colorings, salt, and sugar. If you've been consuming too many fast foods, convenience foods, and junk foods, a raw foods diet could help you dramatically reduce your intake of cholesterol, sugar, saturated fats, and sodium.

Because raw foods diets are low in calories, saturated fat, sugar, and sodium, they may also help you shed unwanted pounds.

> **Food for Thought**
> *Since the raw food movement is relatively new, the debate over whether it's truly beneficial or unnecessary is still going on. Some believe that cooking certain foods makes certain nutrients easier to digest and absorb, and also destroys germs—so why eat them raw?*

As with a standard vegan diet, care must be taken on a raw foods diet to supplement nutrients that may be missing or consumed in inadequate amounts, namely, vitamins B12 and D, iron, and calcium.

While raw foods diets certainly won't have you sweating over a hot stove, they rely on a variety of time-consuming preparation techniques to add different tastes and textures to their meals, including juicing fresh fruits and vegetables; sprouting nuts, seeds, and grains; soaking nuts and dried fruits; blending foods; and dehydrating produce combined with other ingredients to make crackers or other foods.

Going on a raw foods diet can also be expensive, especially if you need to invest in basic equipment like a juicer, blender, dehydrator, and food processor. In addition, many raw foods recipes incorporate costly ingredients found only in health food stores or by mail-order. If you are interested in continuing a raw foods diet after completely the 10-day detox, research your concerns and get in touch with a nutritionist to make sure it's the right diet for you.

Meal Plans for 10-Day Raw Foods Detox

If you tried the Vegan Detox plan and liked it, this may be a natural next step! A large component of this plan involves consuming sprouted grains, seeds, and nuts, which are densely nutritious young versions of the plant. With a little practice, you can grow sprouts at home. Check out *www.real-foods.net/grow-sprouts.html* for an easy tutorial.

Day 1

Breakfast

1 serving Blueberry-Blast Smoothie (page 39)
1 small handful Raw Walnuts
Herbal Tea

Lunch

2 cups Mixed Wild Greens with Chopped Vegetables; Avocado, Lemon, and Extra-virgin Olive Oil; and Raw Sunflower Seeds
8 ounces Fresh Carrot Juice

Dinner

2 Tacos (Stuff purple cabbage leaves with fresh guacamole, tomatoes, and sprouts.)
2 ounces Sprouted Grain Crackers with Fresh Salsa
Herbal Tea

Day 2

Breakfast

8 ounces Fresh Organic Veggie Juice
1 cup Melon or Papaya Slices
1 small handful Sprouted Almonds
Herbal Tea

Lunch

Garden Salad
1½ cups Kiwi Mango Juice (4 kiwifruit, peeled; 3 mangos, pitted; juice together)
1 serving Marinated Kale and Avocado Salad (page 40)
2 ounces Flax or Sprouted Grain Crackers
Freshly Squeezed Lemonade

Dinner

1 cup Sprout Salad with Sunflower Seed Pâté (Sprout sunflower seeds for 2 days; mix with celery, onion, bit of lemon juice, and seasonings in food processor until smooth. Olive oil may be drizzled in to assist with processing.)
1 cup Miso Soup
Vegetable Sticks Marinated in Asian-Flavored Vinaigrette
1 cup Fruit Salad with Lime Juice and Shredded Coconut
Herbal Tea

Meal Plans for 10-Day Raw Foods Detox

Day 3

Breakfast
1 serving Basic Green Smoothie with Pears (page 41)
1 cup Fresh Sliced Bananas with Strawberries
Herbal Tea

Lunch
Leafy Green Salad of Celery, Tomatoes, and Bell Peppers with Olive Oil Dressing
Fresh Berries with Coconut Cream (cream can be made by juicing coconut meat)
8 ounces Water

Dinner
Spinach Salad with Sunflower Seeds and Tahini Dressing
Fresh Vegetable Juice
"Banana split" with Cashew Cream, Strawberries, and Walnuts
Herbal Tea

Day 4

Breakfast
Melon Topped with Berries
½ cup Sprouted Buckwheat Cereal with Almond Milk (Soak buckwheat groats in water overnight, drain and sprout for 2 days, then dehydrate until crispy at temperature below 118°F.)
Herbal Tea

Lunch
Leafy Green Salad with Nuts, Avocadoes, and Orange Juice Dressing
3 Celery Stalks Stuffed with Raw Cashew Butter and Raisins
Water with Orange Slices

Dinner
Spinach Salad with Cucumber, Tomato, Green Onion, and Tahini Garlic Dressing
1 serving Stuffed Red Bell Peppers (page 42)
Herbal Tea

Day 5

Breakfast
Orange-Grapefruit Salad with Sliced Almonds
Strawberry Smoothie
Herbal Tea

Lunch
Cabbage Salad with Nuts, Raisins, and Tahini Dressing with Agave Syrup
Sliced Tomatoes with Olive Oil, Basil, and Sea Salt
Water Flavored with Cucumber Slices

Dinner
1 or 2 Collard Green Burrito Wraps with Cilantro, Tomatoes, and Mexican Pâté (page 43)
1 cup Diced Oranges and Jicama with Lime Juice and Chili Seasoning
16 ounces Watermelon Juice
Herbal Tea

Meal Plans for 10-Day Raw Foods Detox

Breakfast

Sprouted Buckwheat Cereal with Berries and Almond Milk

1 cup Fresh Grapefruit Sections

Herbal Tea

Lunch

1 serving Gazpacho (page 44)

1 cup Mango Pineapple Smoothie (almond milk blended with mango, pineapple, and agave if needed)

2 ounces Raw Corn Chips (Process 5 cups fresh corn, ½ c flax meal, 3 tablespoons lemon juice and spread out in a ¼ inch layer. Dehydrate at low temp until crispy.)

Filtered Water with Lime Slices

Dinner

2 medium Tomatoes Stuffed with Fresh Corn, Cilantro, Jalapeño, Red Bell Pepper, Cucumber, Red Onion, Lime Juice, Olive Oil, Sea Salt

1 cup Baby Spring Greens with Tahini Garlic Dressing

½ cup Lemon Pudding (Blend avocado, lemon juice and zest, and agave syrup.)

Herbal Tea

Breakfast

Almond Banana Milkshake (Blend almond milk with frozen banana and agave to taste.)

Muesli with Nuts and Berries

Herbal Tea

Lunch

Sprouted Sunflower-Carrot-Celery "Burgers" with Basil and Parsley (Process sunflower seeds, carrot, celery, basil, and parsley. Form into patties and dehydrate at low temp until warm.)

Spinach Salad with Marinated Mushrooms

1 cup Organic Veggie Juice

Water

Dinner

1 serving Corn Chowder (page 45)

1 ounce Flax Crackers

Shredded Zucchini with Apples, Avocado, and Cumin

1 Vegan Chocolate Chip Cookie

Herbal Tea

Breakfast

1 cup Citrus-Berry Smoothie with Orange Juice, Strawberries, and Blueberries

1 handful Raw Walnuts

Herbal Tea

Lunch

1½ cups Sprouted Quinoa Tabbouleh with Parsley, Tomatoes, Cucumbers, Red Peppers, Onions, and Lemon Garlic Vinaigrette (Soak quinoa for 1 hour, then sprout for 24–48 hours.)

2 ounces Flax Crackers

1 cup fresh Red and Green Apple Juice

Herbal Tea

Dinner

1 serving Raw Pasta with Tomato Marinara (page 46)

Spinach Salad with Pesto Dressing

Flax Crackers with Almond Butter

1 Frozen Banana

Herbal Tea

Meal Plans for 10-Day Raw Foods Detox

Day 9

Breakfast
Banana-Peach Smoothie
  with Mint
Sprouted Date-Raisin Bread
  with Almond Butter
Herbal Tea

Lunch
½ cup Zucchini Hummus
  (page 47)
2 ounces Flax Crackers
½ cup sliced Carrots and
  Hummus
1 cup sliced Peaches with
  Almond Cream
Filtered Water with Lime
  Slices

Dinner
½ cup Mock Tuna Pâté
  (made from soaked
  almonds and sunflower
  seeds) in a Romaine Let-
  tuce Wrap with Tomatoes,
  Avocados, and Olives
Leafy Green Salad with
  Oranges and Pine Nut
  Dressing
Fresh Strawberry and
  Banana " Ice Cream"
  (Freeze fruit and process
  until creamy.)
Herbal Tea

Day 10

Breakfast
1 cup Basic Green Smoothie
  with Pears (page 41)
Muesli with Berries and Nuts
Herbal Tea

Lunch
1 serving Arugula with
  Strawberries and Hazel-
  nuts (page 48)
Raw Hummus on Flax
  Crackers
Frozen Peach-Strawberry
  Sorbet
Filtered Water with Lemon
  Slices

Dinner
2 cups Taco Salad, with
  Romaine Lettuce, Mexican
  Pâté (page 43), Salsa, and
  Guacamole
Raw Apple-Cranberry Sauce
  with Dates and Walnuts
  (Blend 2 cups apples with
  ½ cup fresh cranberries
  and 4 dates. Stir in ¼ cup
  chopped walnuts.)
Herbal Tea

Blueberry-Blast Smoothie

Serves: 2

INGREDIENTS

2 medium bananas, peeled

6 ounces blueberries

⅛ cup cream of coconut

1 cup fresh pressed apple juice

3 ice cubes

Place bananas and blueberries in blender. Blend.

Add cream of coconut, apple juice, and ice cubes. Blend until smooth.

388 calories | 14 g fat | 62 g carbohydrates | 3 g protein | 9 mg sodium | 3 g fiber

Coconut in a Nutshell

Coconut is high in fiber. Like other nuts, it's also packed with B vitamins, zinc, and iron. Although it contains more saturated fat than any other fruit or veggie, the small amount used in this recipe won't tip the scales.

Marinated Kale and Avocado Salad

Serves: 2

INGREDIENTS

1 bunch dinosaur kale (approximately 3 cups kale)

Salt to taste

2 tablespoons lemon juice

2 tablespoons olive oil

1 tablespoon nama shoyu

1½ cups diced avocado

1 cup cherry tomatoes, chopped

1 tablespoon dulse flakes

Why is Kale a Superfood?

Kale is a vegetable in the cabbage family. It is very strong and hearty and will grow in all soil types and most climates. It is considered a superfood because of the high quantity of concentrated nutrients including carotenoids and other antioxidants, iron, and calcium.

Peel the stems off the kale leaves. (You can compost the stems.) Roll the leaves and chop into small pieces.

Place the chopped kale into a bowl and sprinkle with salt. Massage the salt into the kale by hand and let it sit for 10 minutes so the kale will become soft and wilt.

Pour the lemon juice onto the kale and let it marinate for a few minutes. The acidic lemon juice will further wilt the kale.

Pour the olive oil and nama shoyu onto the kale and mix well.

Top the kale with avocado, chopped cherry tomatoes, and dulse flakes. Enjoy as a side salad with your entree of choice.

378 calories | 31 g fat | 7 g protein | 598 mg sodium | 12 g fiber

Recipes for 10-Day Raw Foods Detox

Basic Green Smoothie with Pears

Serves: 2

INGREDIENTS

4 cups fresh pear

6 tablespoons lemon juice

2 cups water

4 cups lettuce

1 tablespoon mint (optional)

The Great Green Smoothie

The concept of blending leafy greens was popularized by raw food pioneers Ann Wigmore and Victoria Boutenko. Greens are high in protein, chlorophyll, and minerals.

Place pears, lemon juice, and water into the blender. Blend for a short time until ingredients are mixed well.

Gradually add in the lettuce and continue blending until smooth. Add the chopped mint last and pulse until blended. If you blend herbs such as mint for too long, they become bitter.

213 calories | 1 g fat | 3 g protein | 16 mg sodium | 12 g fiber

Stuffed Red Bell Peppers

Serves: 2

INGREDIENTS

½ cup pecans

¼ cup hemp or sesame seeds or soaked sunflower seeds

¼ cup chopped red or white onion

1 tablespoon lime juice

½ tablespoon chopped jalapeño pepper

¼–½ teaspoon salt

½–1 teaspoon Mexican seasoning

2 red bell peppers

½ cup avocado

2 tablespoons cilantro

In a food processor, process the pecans, seeds, onion, lime juice, jalapeño, salt, and seasoning until smooth.

Cut the red bell peppers in half and remove the stems and seeds.

Fill each red bell pepper half full with the pâté and garnish with avocado slices and cilantro.

408 calories | 33 g fat | 12 g protein | 301 mg sodium | 10 g fiber

Mexican Pâté

Serves: 4

INGREDIENTS

2 cups soaked sunflower seeds

1 cup tomato

¼ cup red or white onions

1 cup fresh corn

2 tablespoons lime juice

½ teaspoon oregano

½ teaspoon cumin

½ teaspoon chili powder

¼–½ teaspoon salt

Soak the sunflower seeds for 8 to 12 hours. Drain and rinse.

Dice the tomato and onion. Cut the corn off the cob.

Grind the sunflower seeds in a food processor until smooth. Add the onion, lime juice, oregano, cumin, chili powder, and salt and process until chunky. Add the tomatoes at the very end and pulse briefly.

320 calories | 25 g fat | 12 g protein | 159 mg sodium | 6 g fiber

The Skinny on Sweet Corn

Corn is the most widely grown crop in America. Sometimes called maize, it is a cereal grain that is a staple crop in many cultures throughout the world with uses as both a food and a biofuel. Sweet corn is delicious raw, eaten right off the cob or sliced off the ear and included in vegetable dishes and salads. When making dehydrated crackers or tortillas, frozen corn works better than fresh.

Recipes for 10-Day Raw Foods Detox

Gazpacho

Serves: 4

INGREDIENTS

3 cups tomatoes, diced

2 cups cucumber, peeled and diced

1 cup red bell pepper, diced

1 tablespoon apple cider vinegar

¼ cup onion, diced

1 clove garlic

2 tablespoons olive oil (or sesame or flaxseed oil)

2 tablespoons lemon juice

2 tablespoons fresh chopped basil

2 tablespoons fresh chopped parsley (for garnish)

In a food processor with an S blade, process 2 cups tomato, 1 cup cucumber, ½ cup bell pepper, apple cider vinegar, onion, garlic, olive oil, and lemon juice until well blended but still chunky.

Add the basil and briefly pulse the food processor.

Pour the soup into a bowl and mix with the remaining diced vegetables. Cover the bowl and place in the refrigerator for 2 hours to chill.

Pour into soup bowls and garnish with parsley and optional diced vegetables

113 calories | 7 g fat | 2 g protein | 12 mg sodium | 3 g fiber

What's Behind Gazpacho?

The recipe for gazpacho originated in Spain. This raw vegetable soup is usually served cold in the summertime. It is especially delicious when tomatoes are in season.

Corn Chowder

Serves: 4

INGREDIENTS

1 cup walnuts

1 cup zucchini

¼ cup celery

2 cups corn

1 cup raw Macadamia nuts

2–4 tablespoons olive oil

¼ teaspoon cayenne pepper powder

2 tablespoons agave nectar

½ clove garlic

½ teaspoon salt

3 cups water

2 tablespoons fresh thyme

Soak the walnuts in warm water (boiled water cooled) for 1 to 2 hours. This sweetens the walnuts and brings them to life.

Cut the zucchini into 1½-inch cubes. Dice celery sticks into small pieces. Cut the kernels off four fresh ears of corn.

Create the soup base by blending the Macadamia nuts, walnuts, olive oil, cayenne, agave nectar, garlic, salt, and water.

Pour the soup base into a large bowl and stir in the corn, zucchini, celery, and thyme.

596 calories | 52 g fat | 10 g protein | 317 mg sodium | 8 g fiber

What is Chowder?

A chowder is a thick, rich, and creamy soup. It is commonly made with potatoes and seafood. There is a variation called Manhattan Chowder, which is a red soup base made with tomato. This raw chowder uses nuts for the cream and zucchini replaces the potatoes.

Raw Pasta with Tomato Marinara

Serves: 2

INGREDIENTS

¼ cup soaked or marinated sun-dried tomatoes

1 cup fresh tomatoes

½ cup red bell pepper

2–4 tablespoons minced onion

½–1 clove garlic

1–2 tablespoons olive oil

1 tablespoon minced fresh parsley

1 tablespoon minced basil

½ tablespoon oregano

2 cups zucchini noodles

¼ cup raw olives

Smart Substitution

If you use store-bought marinated sun-dried tomatoes, this takes about 15 minutes. In place of the parsley, basil, and oregano, you can substitute other spices you may have on hand.

Soak the sun-dried tomatoes in a half cup of water for 1 hour. Set aside the zucchini and olives.

In a blender, blend all remaining ingredients until smooth. Blend the fresh herbs last. Add the sun-dried tomato soak water if you need more liquid.

Process the zucchini into noodles using a spiral slicer. Alternatively, use a mandolin or a knife to create long, thin slices.

Place the zucchini noodles in a serving bowl and place a scoop of the tomato sauce on top. Garnish with olives and a sprig of parsley.

150 calories | 9 g fat | 4 g protein | 304 mg sodium | 5 g fiber

Zucchini Hummus

Serves: 4

INGREDIENTS

2 cups zucchini

1–2 cloves garlic

4 tablespoons tahini

2 tablespoons lemon juice

2 tablespoons olive oil

1 teaspoon paprika

1–2 tablespoons parsley

Peel the skin off the zucchini.

Set aside the paprika and parsley. In a food processor with the S blade, process all the other ingredients until smooth.

Place in a serving bowl and garnish with the paprika and parsley.

160 calories | 14 g fat | 4 g protein | 19 mg sodium | 2 g fiber

Recipes for 10-Day Raw Foods Detox

Arugula with Strawberries and Hazelnuts

Serves: 2

INGREDIENTS

1 cup cucumber

1 cup hazelnuts

1 cup strawberries

3 tablespoons olive oil

3 tablespoons lime juice

¼ teaspoon cayenne pepper powder

3 cups arugula

The Mighty Arugula

Arugula, also called rocket, is a leafy green vegetable with a strong, slightly bitter flavor. It is a great source of vitamins A, C, and K, folate, calcium, iron, and magnesium.

Slice the cucumber into thin rounds.

Blend the strawberries into a dressing in the blender. Gradually add the olive oil, lime juice, and cayenne pepper.

Place a bed of arugula on the bottom of a salad bowl. Arrange the cucumber slices on the arugula and garnish with hazelnuts.

Drizzle the dressing on top of the salad and serve.

---

648 calories | 62 g fat | 12 g protein | 11 mg sodium | 9 g fiber

Chapter 4

15-Day Mediterranean Detox

IF YOU'RE BATTLING HIGH CHOLESTEROL, HAVE HEART PROBLEMS, ARE OVER-WEIGHT, or have type-2 diabetes, the Mediterranean Detox Diet could help you lose weight, reduce your risks of heart disease, and help you control your diabetes without medication. Revolving around fruits and vegetables, whole grains, monounsaturated fats like canola and olive oils, fish, and limited amounts of meat, the Mediterranean Detox is high in fiber and disease-fighting antioxidants and phytochemicals. It's also so delicious and filling that you'll forget you're on a detox diet.

A Breakdown of the Mediterranean Diet

The Mediterranean diet is basically a plant-based diet, which means you eat less meat than you'd consume on the SAD, and get most of your daily protein from plant sources like beans, nuts, and fish.

For years, scientists were baffled by the "French paradox," or why the French, Italians, and Greeks enjoy a lower risk of heart disease, obesity, and stroke than Americans although they consume a diet high in fats, bread, and wine. Today, they understand why: the Mediterranean Diet is low in animal protein, saturated fats, and cholesterol, and high in heart-healthy unsaturated fats like beans, nuts, and fish.

Far less restrictive than the raw foods or vegan diets, the Mediterranean Detox is comprised of everyday foods that most Americans already enjoy. You won't have to invest in expensive equipment, stalk health food stores for exotic ingredients, or heat your evening meal in a Mr. Coffee, like on the raw food diet. Here are some other reasons you may enjoy eating like the French, Greeks, and Italians.

You'll consume wholesome, delicious, and satisfying meals that bear no resemblance to diet or detox fare. A Mediterranean diet revolves around fruits, vegetables, pasta, and rice, with just a touch of animal protein. For instance, the Greeks eat very little red meat and average nine servings of produce daily.

You won't have to give up healthy fats. On the Mediterranean Detox, you replace artery-clogging saturated fats found in animal protein with unsaturated fats found in plants, including olive, sesame, and canola oils; walnuts; pecans; almonds; and hazelnuts. Unsaturated fats are also high in omega-3 fatty acids, which lower triglyceride levels and improve the health of blood vessels, which in turn helps reduce the incidence of heart disease and stroke.

You won't have to give up bread. The Mediterranean Detox includes ample portions of whole-grain breads and pastas, which contain very few unhealthy saturated or trans fats. But you'll eat your carbs like a Mediterranean, not like an American. Instead of slathering your bread and pasta with butter or margarine, which are high in saturated fats, you'll enjoy them with olive oil, which contains heart-healthy unsaturated fats.

You won't have to give up all meat. The Mediterranean Detox encourages you to eat fish at least twice a week, consume chicken in moderation, and indulge in red meat and pork a few times a month.

You don't have to give up wine. On the Mediterranean Detox, you can enjoy moderate amounts of wine at lunch and dinner. If you are someone who cannot or should not consume alcohol, such as a pregnant woman, you will still gain the same benefits from drinking red grape juice.

You won't have to sacrifice taste. If you've ever eaten French, Italian, or Greek cuisine, you already know that Mediterranean fare is some of the most delicious food on earth.

Food for Thought

Studies show that consuming a Mediterranean diet allowed people with type-2 diabetes to lose weight easier and reduce their risk of cardiovascular disease. The study called the diet "a safe and tasty means to delay the introduction of anti-diabetic drug therapy in newly diagnosed type 2 diabetic people."

Meal Plans for 15-Day Mediterranean Detox Diet

To transition to the heart-healthy Mediterranean diet, all you need to do is focus on reducing red meat consumption and increasing your intake of fish, nuts, vegetables, and olive oil. The occasional glass of red wine is also encouraged! For Days 8–15, go to Day 1 and repeat the sequence.

Breakfast

1 cup Couscous with Dried Fruit (page 54)
2 Scrambled Eggs with Feta Cheese and Spinach
Herbal Tea or Coffee

Lunch

1 cup Gazpacho
2 Garlic Breadsticks
1 small Fruit and Cheese Plate
HerbalTea

Dinner

5 ounces Baked Chicken with Olives and Tomatoes (page 55)
1 cup Chunky Greek Salad (page 56)
1 Dinner Roll
1 baked Phyllo Cup with Berries and Honey
Herbal Tea or 1 glass Red Wine (optional)

Day 1

Breakfast

2-Egg Veggie Omelet (broccoli, peppers, onions, mushrooms, etc.)
1 slice Whole-Grain Toast with Jam
6 ounces Fresh Orange Juice with Pulp
Herbal Tea or Coffee

Lunch

1 cup Blood Orange Salad with Shrimp (page 57)
1 cup White Bean Soup with Shredded Kale, Lemon, Garlic
½ cup Fresh Melons
Herbal Tea

Dinner

1½ cups Mediterranean Seafood Soup (page 58)
½ cup Garlicky Sautéed Greens
1 Crusty Dinner Roll
1 cup Berries with Yogurt and Sunflower Seeds
Herbal Tea or 1 glass Red Wine (optional)

Day 2

Breakfast

1 cup Hot Multigrain Cereal
1 cup Mixed Fruit with Greek-Style Yogurt and Honey
Herbal Tea

Lunch

1 Lemony Tuna Salad in Pita Bread
1 cup Vegetable Lentil Soup
Herbal Tea

Dinner

1 cup Spinach Salad with Mushrooms, Radishes, Olive Oil, and Balsamic Vinegar
1 cup Quinoa with Chick Peas and Fresh Herbs
¾ cup Strawberry Banana Sundae
Herbal Tea or 1 glass Red Wine (optional)

Day 3

Meal Plans for 15-Day Mediterranean Detox Diet

Day 4

Breakfast
6 ounces Orange Juice
2-Egg Omelet with
  Vegetables
1 cup Fresh Berries with
  Greek-Style Yogurt
Herbal Tea

Lunch
1 cup Italian Seafood Salad
  (page 59)
1 Pita Bread with Hummus
Herbal Tea

Dinner
½ cup Ratatouille
4 ounces Grilled Herbed
  Chicken
1 cup Green Salad
½ cup Vanilla Bean Ice
  Cream with Chopped Date
  and Nut Topping
Herbal Tea or 1 glass Red
  Wine (optional)

Day 5

Breakfast
1 Hard-Boiled Egg
1 slice Whole Wheat Toast
½ cup Greek-Style Yogurt
  with Honey and Nuts
Herbal Tea

Lunch
1 cup Minestrone Soup
  (page 60)
1 Pita with Hummus, Tomato,
  Cucumber, and Onion
Herbal Tea

Dinner
4 ounces Grilled Lamb and
  Vegetable Kebobs
½ cup Rice Pilaf with Fresh
  Herbs
1 Grilled Pear with Whipped
  Topping
Herbal Tea or 1 glass Red
  Wine (optional)

Day 6

Breakfast
¾ cup Granola with 1 cup
  Milk
½ cup Mixed Fruit Salad
Herbal Tea

Lunch
5 ounces Roasted Cod with
  Fresh Salsa (page 61)
1 cup Creamy Cauliflower
  Soup
1 piece Crusty Bread
Herbal Tea

Dinner
1½ cups Pasta with Grilled
  Shrimp, Lemon, Garlic,
  Olive Oil, Parsley
1 cup Roasted Mixed Bell
  Peppers with Olive Oil and
  Garlic
1 Baked Apple
Herbal Tea or 1 glass Red
  Wine (optional)

Meal Plans for 15-Day Mediterranean Detox Diet

Breakfast

1 cup Fruit and Yogurt
   Smoothie
2 cinnamon Phyllo Crisps
Herbal Tea

Lunch

1 Falafel Pita Sandwich with
   Lettuce, Tomato, and
   Tahini Dressing
1 cup Cucumber and Carrot
   Sticks with Hummus
Herbal Tea

Dinner

5 ounces Snapper Mediter-
   ranean Style (page 62)
½ grilled Artichoke with
   Olive Oil, Lemon, and
   Herbs
1 cup Green Salad
1 slice Ricotta Cheesecake
   (page 63)
Herbal Tea or 1 glass Red
   Wine (optional)

Couscous with Dried Fruit

Serves: 4

INGREDIENTS

1 cup vegetable broth

½ teaspoon kosher salt

½ teaspoon cinnamon

3 tablespoons olive oil

1 cup couscous

3 tablespoons dried apricots, chopped

3 tablespoons dried cherries, chopped

3 tablespoons craisins, chopped

3 tablespoons Italian parsley, minced

Bring broth, salt, cinnamon, and olive oil to a boil. Stir in the couscous and dried fruit.

Return to boil. Cover and remove from heat.

Let stand for 5 minutes. Fluff with fork and stir in parsley.

336 calories | 12.3 g fat | 49.57 g carbohydrate | 6.5 g protein | 746 mg sodium | 1.2 g fiber

Why Are Cherries for Good for Gout?

Dried cherries contain concentrated doses of the same nutrients found in raw ones. Along with antioxidants, cherries contain keracyanin, a coloring pigment believed to lower high blood levels of uric acid and relieve symptoms of gout.

Baked Chicken with Olives and Tomatoes

Serves: 2

INGREDIENTS

8 ounces organic boneless skinless chicken breasts

1 tablespoon Greek oregano

½ pound mushrooms, sliced

3 tablespoon extra-virgin olive oil, divided

1 large garlic clove, minced

⅓ cup dry white wine

¼ cup dry sherry

2 large Roma tomatoes, seeded and cut into small cubes

2 tablespoons tomato paste

¼ cup pitted kalamata olives, sliced

A Minute for Mushrooms

The lowly mushroom is loaded with potassium (even more than bananas) and can help lower cholesterol. One serving of mushrooms also provides up to 40 percent of the RDA for copper, which helps protect the heart. Mushrooms are also high in riboflavin, niacin, and selenium, which helps protect against the damaging effects of free radicals.

Rinse chicken under cold water. Pat dry and season with Greek oregano.

Sauté mushrooms in 1 tablespoon olive oil until brown. Add garlic and cook for 1 minute.

Remove mushrooms from pan. Add 2 tablespoons olive oil and sear chicken breasts. Remove chicken from pan and place in baking dish coated with cooking spray.

Add wine and sherry to pan. Stir in tomatoes, tomato paste, mushrooms, and garlic. Cook until the sauce thickens.

Place black olives on top of chicken and pour tomato sauce on top.

Cover pan with foil and bake in 350°F oven for 45 minutes. The sauce will thicken as it bakes.

488 calories | 29.6 g fat | 15.33 g carbohydrate | 31.8 g protein | 647 mg sodium | 2.2 g fiber

Chunky Greek Salad

Serves: 2

INGREDIENTS

1 cucumber, peeled

2 Roma tomatoes, sliced

¼ cup red onion, diced

⅛ cup pitted kalamata olives, sliced

3 tablespoons fresh lemon juice.

½ teaspoon dried oregano.

3 tablespoons extra-virgin olive oil.

Salt and pepper to taste

⅛ cup feta cheese, crumbled

3 tablespoons Italian parsley, minced

Mix cucumbers, tomatoes, red onion, and olives together.

For dressing, mix lemon juice, oregano, and olive oil together in a small jar. Shake vigorously.

Toss lemon juice dressing over cucumber mixture.

Add salt and pepper to taste.

Place salad on plates and sprinkle with feta and parsley.

296 calories | 24 g fat | 15 g carbohydrate | 4 g protein | 548 mg sodium | 2.1 g fiber

Onions for Achoo?

Got a cold or the flu? Onions can help eliminate mucus in the upper respiratory tract, and also act as disinfectants in the body, so don't overlook them when you're under the weather.

Blood Orange Salad with Shrimp

Serves: 4

INGREDIENTS

2 bags baby spinach (try to find prewashed)

2 blood oranges

1¼ pounds chilled, cooked shrimp, peeled

Juice of ½ lemon

¼ cup extra-virgin olive oil

¼ teaspoon dry mustard

Salt and pepper to taste

¼ cup stemmed, loosely packed parsley or cilantro (whichever you like)

Just before serving, place the spinach on individual serving plates.

Peel the oranges. Slice them crossways, about ¼-inch thick, picking out any seeds. Arrange on top of the spinach. Arrange the shrimp around the oranges.

Place the rest of the ingredients in the blender and puree until the dressing is a bright green. Pour over the salads.

Serve chilled.

314 calories | 16 g fat | 14 g carbohydrates | 32 g protein | 386 mg sodium | 1 g fiber

Why Are Blood Oranges Red?

Blood oranges are a type of orange with crimson-colored flesh. The "blood" color comes from the presence of anthocyanin, a pigment that's found in many other fruits and flowers, but not usually in oranges. Like regular oranges, blood oranges are high in vitamins C, B, K, biotin, folic acid, amino acids, and minerals. They help cleanse the gastro-intestinal track, and lower high blood pressure.

Mediterranean Seafood Soup

Serves: 2

INGREDIENTS

2 tablespoons olive oil

½ cup sweet onion, chopped

2 cloves garlic, chopped

½ bulb fennel, chopped

½ cup dry white wine

1 cup clam broth (canned is fine)

2 cups tomatoes, chopped

6 littleneck clams, tightly closed

6 mussels, tightly closed

8 raw jumbo shrimp, peeled and deveined

1 teaspoon dried basil or 5 leaves fresh basil, torn

Salt and red pepper flakes to taste

Heat the oil over medium flame and add onion, garlic, and fennel. After 10 minutes, stir in the wine and clam broth and add the tomatoes. Bring to a boil.

Drop clams into the boiling liquid. When clams start to open, add the mussels. When mussels start to open, add the shrimp, basil, salt, and pepper flakes. Serve when shrimp turns pink.

450 calories | 18 g fat | 19 g carbohydrate | 48 g protein | 1,162 mg sodium | 1.7 g fiber

The Low-Down on Littleneck Clams

Littleneck clams are the smallest variety of hard-shell clams and can be found on the northern east and west coasts of the United States. They have a sweet taste and are delicious steamed and dipped in melted butter, battered and fried, or baked.

Italian Seafood Salad

Serves: 4

INGREDIENTS

¼ cup water

¼ cup dry white wine

1 teaspoon lemon juice

16 medium raw shrimp, peeled and deveined

16 medium sea scallops

½ pound fillet of skinless bluefish, turbot, scrod, or halibut

1 pound cracked Alaskan crab legs, cut in 2-inch lengths

½ pound mussels, scrubbed

1 cup light or low-fat Italian dressing

2 teaspoons capers

Black pepper to taste

1 cup fresh Italian flat-leaf parsley, pulled from stems

½ teaspoon coriander seeds, cracked

1 teaspoon lemon zest

12 tiny currant tomatoes

½ red onion, thinly sliced

Set a large bowl next to the stove. In a large pot, mix together the water, wine, and lemon juice; bring to a boil. Poach the shrimp and sea scallops for 5 minutes and then remove to the bowl. Place the bluefish, turbot, scrod, or halibut into the pot and allow to simmer for 4 minutes. Remove and add to the bowl of seafood. Drop the crab leg pieces into the boiling liquid. Remove after 1 minute. Place in the bowl.

Poach the mussels until they are open. Place in the bowl.

Add to the bowl the Italian dressing and the rest of the ingredients. Toss gently to coat. Refrigerate for 2 hours. Serve chilled or at room temperature.

553 calories | 33 g fat | 6 g carbohydrate | 58 g protein | 2,947 mg sodium | .65 g fiber

Why is Wine So Wonderful?

Wine contains disease-fighting phytochemicals that help decrease the risk of heart disease and certain cancers and slow the progression of neurological degenerative diseases like Alzheimer's and Parkinson's. But don't drink more than two glasses a day, or your health benefits will go down the drain. Remember, red grape juice provides the same benefits as red wine.

Minestrone Soup

Serves: 8

INGREDIENTS

3 tablespoons extra-virgin olive oil

1 large carrot, peeled and diced

1 large red bell pepper, diced

1 large white onion, diced

16 ounces can whole tomatoes in juice

2 cups vegetable broth

1 teaspoon dried oregano

2 teaspoons Italian seasoning

½ pound fresh green beans, cut into 1-inch pieces.

½ cup orzo

8 ounces can dark kidney beans, drained and rinsed

1 (15-ounce) can cannellini beans, not drained

1 small zucchini, cut into 1-inch cubes

1 medium Roma tomato, diced

Salt and pepper to taste

6 ounce bag baby spinach

Fresh ground pepper, to taste

1 cup fresh grated Parmesan cheese

In a large soup pot heat oil and sauté carrots, bell pepper, and onion. Cook over medium heat for 2 minutes.

Drain canned tomatoes and reserve juice. Add to vegetables.

Add vegetable broth and spices. Bring to a boil and lower heat to simmer.

Add green beans, kidney beans, cannellini beans, zucchini, diced Roma tomato, and orzo.

Simmer until orzo is soft.

Season with salt and pepper. Add the spinach and cook until it is wilted.

Pour into bowls and garnish with freshly ground pepper and Parmesan cheese.

378 calories | 5 g fat | 59 g carbohydrates | 23 g protein | 657 mg sodium | 5 g fiber

What Is Orzo?

Orzo is a type of Italian pasta that is shaped like rice, only larger. Made of semolina, it is a close relative of couscous, and can be used interchangeably with couscous, rice, barley, and other grains, in many dishes.

Recipes for 15-Day Mediterranean Detox Diet

Roasted Cod with Fresh Salsa

Serves: 2

INGREDIENTS

12 ounces fresh cod, rinsed

1 tablespoon extra-virgin olive oil

½ teaspoon kosher salt and black pepper

½ cup kalamata olives, sliced in half

1 Roma tomato, seeded and chopped

¼ red onion, finely diced

1 garlic clove, minced

1 tablespoon capers

1 teaspoon lemon zest

2 tablespoons fresh lemon juice

4 basil leaves, chiffonade

Brush cod with olive oil and season with salt and pepper.

Prepare salsa by mixing olives, tomato, onion, garlic, capers, lemon zest, and lemon juice.

Grill cod on well-oiled grill for 3–4 minutes per side or until the fish is translucent and is cooked through.

Place cod on plate and top with salsa and basil.

348 calories | 20.8 g fat | 9.3 g carbohydrate | 30.7 g protein | 1,830 mg sodium | 1.9 g fiber

What Is Chiffonade?

Chiffonade is the French word for "little rags." Layer your herb leaves on top of one another and roll them like a miniature cigar. Then slice the "cigar" into pretty chiffonade pieces of herb.

Recipes for 15-Day Mediterranean Detox Diet

Snapper Mediterranean Style

Serves: 2

INGREDIENTS

½ cup minced shallots

2 tablespoon extra-virgin olive oil, divided

¼ cup dry vermouth

Kosher salt and fresh cracked black pepper to taste

12 ounces fresh snapper fillets, rinsed

¼ cup dry white wine

¼ cup red onion, finely diced

½ jalapeño pepper, seeded and diced

1 cup cherry tomatoes, sliced in half

2 ounces green olives, finely diced

2 ounces feta cheese, crumbled

Hot! Hot! Hot!

High in vitamins C and A, all types of red peppers, including the feisty jalapeño (which is red when ripe), stimulate circulation and tone and cleanse the arteries and heart muscle.

Sauté shallot in 1 tablespoon olive oil until very soft.

Add vermouth and reduce this liquid by half.

Season snapper with salt and pepper. Sauté in olive oil shallot mixture. Add white wine. Cover pan and let fish steam until cooked through. Add water or additional white wine if there is not enough liquid to complete cooking the fish.

Combine onion, jalapeño, tomatoes, and olives to form salsa.

Add 1 tablespoon olive oil and season with salt and pepper.

Place fish on warm platter and top fish with salsa and feta cheese.

439 calories | 20 g fat | 16 g carbohydrate | 40 g protein | 1,894 mg sodium | 2 g fiber

Ricotta Cheesecake

Serves: 12

INGREDIENTS

3 tablespoons unsalted butter, melted

1½ cups graham cracker crumbs

24 ounces ricotta cheese

1 cup granulated sugar

2 teaspoons pure vanilla extract

½ cup light sour cream

4 large eggs

The Egg and I

Eggs have gotten an undeserved bad rap. Studies show they provide all nine essential amino acids and may help reduce macular degeneration, cataracts, and—surprise!—heart disease and stroke. Studies showed women who ate six eggs a week lowered their breast cancer risk by 44 percent.

Mix melted butter with graham cracker crumbs. Press into a 10-inch springform pan lined with parchment paper.

Beat ricotta cheese with sugar until very smooth. Add vanilla extract and sour cream.

Beat eggs in one at time. Scrape sides of bowl.

Place ricotta mixture into the cheesecake crust.

Bake at 325°F for 45–55 minutes in a water bath.

Remove from oven and cool. Place in refrigerator for at least 24 hours before unmolding.

Unmold cheesecake by carefully opening the springform pan.

282 calories | 14 g fat | 28 g carbohydrate | 11 g protein | 192 mg sodium | .12 g fiber

Part II

Elimination Detox Diets

The purpose of an elimination detox diet is to remove or reduce substances or toxins from your body that may cause allergic reactions, illnesses, or serious diseases. Elimination diets are often used to determine if an actual intolerance exists and then may be used to help you eliminate or reduce symptoms associated with that intolerance. This chapter covers four elimination diets. The 10-Day Gluten Detox and the 10-Day Lactose Detox target gluten or lactose in your diet. The 5-Day Acid Balance reduces your intake of acidic foods and restores your body's healthy acid/alkaline balance. The 30-Day Heavy Metal Detox revolves around nutrients that displace dangerous environmental toxins lodged in your organs. It helps your body neutralize and eliminate them. These diets are not interchangeable.

Chapter 5

10-Day Gluten Detox

IF YOU'RE ALLERGIC TO GLUTEN, YOU SUFFER FROM CELIAC DISEASE, an intestinal disorder caused by intolerance to gluten, a protein found in wheat, rye, barley, and other grains. Gluten irritates the intestinal lining, interfering with the absorption of nutrients and water. Unlike some allergies, you don't outgrow celiac disease. Once you have it, you must maintain a gluten-free diet to avoid symptoms, which range from bloating, nausea, and diarrhea to potential long-term illness. If you suffer with these symptoms, this 10-day elimination diet can help you determine if gluten may be the culprit.

Coping with Celiac Disease

Many people don't know much about gluten-free diets until they find out they need to be on one. About 1 in 133 people suffer from celiac disease, and health organizations say between 6 and 7 million Americans suffer from food allergies. A great resource for people with this disease is the Celiac Disease Foundation (*www.celiac.org*).

Unlike with other autoimmune diseases, physicians know the trigger for celiac disease: gluten, which provokes an immune response that causes the body to attack itself. Gluten can be found in unlikely places, including:

- Sour cream, ice cream, and cheese
- Nondairy creamers
- Meat patties and sausages
- Soy meat substitutes
- Malt flavoring and caramel coloring
- Rice mixes and seasoning mixes

> **DETOX TIP**
>
> Testing for celiac disease starts with blood work, in which physicians study the series of antibodies that provide a good marker of the tendency to have the illness. Blood work is often followed up with an intestinal biopsy.

- Some medications
- Canned soups and bouillon cubes
- Salad dressing, mustard, flavored vinegars, and mayonnaise
- Canned baked beans and vegetables with sauces
- Nonstick baking sprays with flour
- Cocoa mixes and chocolate drinks

What Can I Eat?

Once you've made the decision to be gluten free, you can purchase ingredients at natural food stores, supermarkets, and online. Fresh fruits, meats, and veggies are a great place to start—always remember, if they are fresh, they are gluten free. If the food is manufactured or prepared, chances are it contains gluten. Avoid pre-seasoned foods, as flour may have been added to the seasoning mix. You should also invest in a few good gluten-free cookbooks.

> **DETOX TIP**
>
> To put together a gluten-free pantry, make sure you have four kinds of flour, including rice, corn, walnut (a sweet flour that works great for desserts), and quinoa, a high-protein flour.

Maintaining a healthy gluten-free lifestyle involves eating a well-balanced diet that is high in protein and moderate in fats. Common nutrient shortages among people with celiac disease include deficiencies in calcium; the vitamin B complex; and vitamins A, C, D, K, and E.

You can make your kitchen a safe place to cook and eat with this four-step approach to clearing out gluten.

1. Remove foods that are unhealthy.
2. Replace these with ingredients that are important for your nutrition.
3. Rejuvenate with exercise and healthy living.
4. Repair your body with a steady and healthy dietary regimen.

In addition, restaurants can be landmines when it comes to gluten-free eating, but with some practice, you can avoid the pitfalls.

- Mentally eliminate the pasta, the sandwiches, the gravy and sauces, and anything that looks complicated.
- Many restaurant sauces have gluten in them, and sometimes the beef and chicken are prepared and vacuum packed in a broth that contains gluten. Some soy sauces may have gluten.

- Ask for your salad without croutons.
- Avoid anything breaded or battered.
- Steer clear of French fries, onion rings, chicken wings, and other foods that have been dusted with flour.

Luckily there are a few food chains that are becoming more accommodating to those with celiac disease. The chains that offer gluten-free menu additions include Outback Steakhouse and P. F. Chang's.

Food for Thought

If you're having trouble coping with your disease or just need some encouragement while you start your new way of eating, talk to friends or support groups who have had experience with celiac disease or food allergies.

Meal Plans for 10-Day Gluten Detox

Sticking to a gluten-free plan is easy once you make the effort to ditch processed foods where gluten normally lurks. But you don't have to give up everything you once loved! Due to the rise in cases of celiac disease, many manufacturers now offer options for gluten-free flours, breads, cake mixes, and more.

Day 1

Breakfast
2 Blueberry and Strawberry Pancakes (page 74)
2 slices Turkey Bacon
Herbal Tea or Coffee

Lunch
2–3 Crab Cakes (made with gluten-free breadcrumbs)
1 cup Salad with Baby Greens and Balsamic Vinaigrette
Herbal Tea

Dinner
4 ounce Herb-Roasted Turkey
½ cup Gluten-Free Rosemary Stuffing
1 cup Spinach Salad with Orange Juice Dressing
Herbal Tea
1 Gluten-Free Chocolate Chip Cookie

Day 2

Breakfast
2 Scrambled Eggs with Gluten-Free Cheese, Onions, and Tomatoes
1 slice Gluten-Free Toast with All-Natural Berry Preserves
6 ounces Freshly Squeezed Orange Juice
Herbal Tea or Coffee

Lunch
1 cup Mixed Greens d with 4-ounces Sliced Steak
1 Gluten-Free Roll
1 cup Yogurt with Fruit
Herbal Tea

Dinner
½ Roasted Cornish Game Hen with Ginger-Orange Glaze (page 75)
½ cup Garlic Mashed Potatoes
1 cup Garden Salad
½ cup Vanilla Ice Cream with Berries

Day 3

Breakfast
1 Spicy Egg and Cheese–Stuffed Tomato (page 76)
1 slice Gluten-Free Toast with Fresh Fruit Preserves
6 ounces Fresh Grapefruit Juice
Herbal Tea

Lunch
1 cup Gluten-Free Pasta Salad with Asparagus
1 cup Spicy Tomato Soup
1 ounce Gluten-Free Tortilla Chips (like Santitas white corn tortilla chips)
Herbal Tea

Dinner
4 ounces Spinach-Garlic Meat Loaf
1/2 cup Roasted New Potatoes
1 cup Garden Salad with Olive Oil Dressing
Herbal Tea
1 slice Ricotta Cheesecake with Berries (page 63)

Meal Plans for 10-Day Gluten Detox

Breakfast

1 cup Oatmeal with Berries and Nuts
2 slices Turkey Bacon
6 ounces Fresh Orange Juice
Herbal Tea

Lunch

1 Sloppy Joe Sandwich in a Gluten-Free Bun
1 serving Chopped Salad (page 77)
½ cup Fresh Fruit
Herbal Tea

Dinner

1 cup Gluten-Free Spaghetti and 3 Homemade Meatballs
1 cup Spinach Salad with Sesame Dressing
1 Gluten-Free Roll
Herbal Tea
1 Gluten-Free Brownie

Breakfast

2 Gluten-Free Breakfast Crepes with Berries
2 ounces Turkey Sausage
½ cup Grapefruit Sections
Herbal Tea

Lunch

1 Bunless Cheeseburger with Fried Onions
½ cup Baked French Fries
½ cup Fresh Fruit
Herbal Tea

Dinner

1 cup Old Southern Brunswick Stew (page 78)
1 cup Brown Rice
1 cup Spinach Salad with Tahini Dressing
Herbal Tea
1 piece Gluten-Free Vanilla Cake (Try Betty Crocker's Gluten Free Box Mix.)

Breakfast

6 ounces Apple Juice
1 Gluten-Free Croissant with Fresh Fruit Preserves
2 slices Turkey Bacon
½ cup Berries Topped with Yogurt
Herbal Tea

Lunch

1 cup Thai Pasta Salad with Gluten-Free Pasta
1 cup Orange Sections Dusted with Cinnamon
Herbal Tea
2 small Oatmeal-Raisin Cookies

Dinner

4 ounces Lemon Ginger Chicken
½ cup Asparagus
1 cup Garden Salad with Tahini Dressing
Herbal Tea
1 serving Panna Cotta (page 79)

Meal Plans for 10-Day Gluten Detox

Day 7

Breakfast

6 ounces Orange Juice
2 Gluten-Free Waffles with Blueberries
2 slices Turkey Bacon
Herbal Tea

Lunch

1½ cups Asian Grilled Chicken Salad (skip the fried wontons)
2 Vegetable Spring Rolls
Herbal Tea

Dinner

4 ounces Roast Beef
1 cup Wild Rice Salad (page 80)
½ cup Steamed Sugar Snap Peas
Herbal Tea
1 slice Gluten-Free Blueberry-Apple Pie

Day 8

Breakfast

6 ounces Apple Juice
1 slice Gluten-Free Chocolate Cake
2 turkey Sausage Patties
½ cup Grapefruit Sections

Lunch

1 cup Minestrone Soup (without pasta or using gluten-free macaroni)
1 Gluten-Free Dinner Roll
½ cup Fresh Fruit
Herbal Tea

Dinner

5 ounces Beef Stroganoff (page 81)
1 cup Buttered Gluten-Free Noodles
½ cup Steamed Asparagus with Lemon
Herbal Tea
¾ cup Banana Pudding with Gluten-Free Vanilla Wafers

Day 9

Breakfast

6 ounces Apple Juice
1 cup Steel-Cut Oatmeal with Nuts and Raisins
½ cup Orange and Grapefruit Sections

Lunch

2 cups Chef Salad with Light Ranch Dressing
½ cup Baked French Fries
Herbal Tea
½ cup Fresh Fruit

Dinner

1 serving Grilled Eggplant Parmesan (page 82)
1 cup Garden Salad with Olive Oil and Balsamic Vinegar Dressing
Herbal Tea
½ cup Vanilla Ice Cream with Hot Fudge Sauce

Meal Plans for 10-Day Gluten Detox

Breakfast

2-Egg Mushroom Spinach Omelet
1 slice Gluten-Free Toast with Fresh Fruit Preserves
½ cup Melon Slices
Herbal Tea

Lunch

1 cup Homemade Roasted Tomato Soup
1 slice Corn Bread
1 cup Spinach Salad with Tahini Dressing
Herbal Tea

Dinner

1 Stuffed Pork Chop (page 83)
1 cup Garden Salad with Olive Oil and Balsamic Vinegar
Herbal Tea
¾ cup Frozen Yogurt with Berry Topping

Recipes for 10-Day Gluten Detox

Blueberry and Strawberry Pancakes

Yields: 12 pancakes

INGREDIENTS

½ cup milk

2 eggs

1½ tablespoons butter, melted

1 tablespoon baking powder

1 cup rice flour (or substitute corn, chickpea, or tapioca flour)

Extra butter for frying pancakes

¼ pint blueberries

¼ pint strawberries

1 tablespoon sugar

1 teaspoon orange zest

Bring on the Pancakes!

Think you can't have pancakes because you're allergic to wheat? Think again! The rice flour subs nicely for wheat flour. Blueberries also contain saponins, which improve heart health, and the strawberries provide potassium, which is essential for immune system function and for strong connective tissue.

In the bowl of a food processor whirl the milk, eggs, and melted butter. Slowly add the baking powder and flour.

Heat griddle pan or large frying pan to medium. Drop a teaspoon of butter on it and when the butter sizzles, start pouring on the batter to about 2 inches in diameter.

When bubbles come to the top, turn the pancakes and continue to fry until golden brown. Place on a plate in a warm oven to keep warm while you make the others.

In a bowl, mix the fruit, sugar, and orange zest. Mash with potato masher or pestle.

---

90 calories | 2.7 g fat | 14 g carbohydrate | 2.2 g protein | 114 mg sodium | .2 g fiber

Recipes for 10-Day Gluten Detox

Roasted Cornish Game Hens with Ginger-Orange Glaze

Serves: 4

INGREDIENTS
2 Cornish game hens, split
2 tablespoons olive oil
Generous sprinkle of salt and pepper
1 tablespoon orange marmalade
2 tablespoons peanut oil
1 tablespoon wheat-free soy sauce
2 tablespoons orange juice
1 tablespoon minced fresh gingerroot

A Spice with Kick

Ginger is a potent detoxer. It has antibacterial and antifungal properties that help aid digestion, break down proteins, and lower high blood pressure by stimulating circulation. Ginger also helps lower LDL, "bad" cholesterol.

Preheat oven to 375°F.

Rinse hens, pat dry with paper towels, brush with olive oil, and sprinkle with salt and pepper.

Stir the rest of the ingredients together in a small saucepan over low heat to make glaze; set aside.

Roast hens in a baking dish or pan, cut side up, for 15 minutes. Turn hens and brush with glaze. Continue to roast for another 20 minutes, brushing hens with glaze every 5 minutes.

---

683 calories | 52.65 g fat | 4.5 g carbohydrate |
47.6 g protein | 662 mg sodium | 0.1 g fiber

Recipes for 10-Day Gluten Detox

Spicy Egg and Cheese–Stuffed Tomatoes

Serves: 4

INGREDIENTS

8 medium tomatoes

2 cloves garlic, minced or pressed

4 tablespoons butter

1 teaspoon salt

1 teaspoon black pepper

1 teaspoon cayenne pepper

1 teaspoon dried oregano

1 teaspoon cumin powder

8 eggs

½ cup grated Monterey jack or Cheddar cheese

8 teaspoons gluten-free cornbread crumbs

Why Tomatoes Help Reduce Cancer

Tomatoes are high in lycopene, which has anti-cancer properties, as well as vitamin C and potassium, which cleanse the liver and help stimulate circulation.

Cut the tops off the tomatoes, core, and use a melon baller to scoop out seeds and pulp. Place the tomatoes on a baking sheet covered with parchment paper or sprayed with nonstick spray.

Preheat the oven to 350°F.

Sauté the garlic in the butter. While it's cooking, mix together the salt, black pepper, cayenne pepper, oregano, and cumin in a small bowl.

Rub the insides of the tomatoes with the spice mixture, saving a bit aside for the eggs. Spoon the butter and garlic mixture into the tomatoes. Sprinkle ½ of the remaining spice mixture.

Break an egg into each tomato. Sprinkle the rest of the spice mixture. Loosely spoon the cheese over the eggs, then sprinkle 1 teaspoon cornbread crumbs over each tomato. Bake for 20 minutes. The tomatoes should still be firm, the eggs soft, the cheese melted, and the bread crumbs browned.

379 calories | 26.7 g fat | 15.7 g carbohydrate | 18.8 g protein | 931 mg sodium | 1.8 g fiber

Chopped Salad

Serves: 4

INGREDIENTS

1 large head of romaine, chopped

1 large cucumber, peeled and diced

1 (15-ounce) can low-sodium garbanzo beans, drained and rinsed

1 medium green onion, diced

2 medium Roma tomatoes, seeded and diced

3 tablespoons fresh lemon juice

1 tablespoon honey

Salt and pepper to taste

¼ cup extra-virgin olive oil

¼ cup feta cheese, crumbled

Fresh ground black pepper

In large bowl combine lettuce, cucumber, garbanzo beans, green onion, and tomato.

Mix lemon juice with honey and salt and pepper. Whisk in olive oil.

Add dressing to bowls of vegetables and beans.

Serve on cold salad plates and top with feta and freshly ground black pepper.

---

235 calories | 17 g fat | 11 g carbohydrate | 8 g protein | 269 mg sodium | 1 g fiber

Lettuce Begin

Romaine lettuce is a good source of calcium, chlorophyll, iron, magnesium, potassium silicon, and vitamins A and E. It helps rebuild hemoglobin, adds shine and thickness to hair, and promotes hair growth.

Old Southern Brunswick Stew

Serves: 6

INGREDIENTS

1 chicken (4 to 5 pounds), cut into serving pieces

⅓ cup rice flour

2 tablespoons butter

1 cup water

2 cups chopped tomatoes, fresh or canned

1 medium onion, chopped

1 cup lima beans

1 cup corn kernels

4 whole cloves of garlic

1 tablespoon gluten-free Worcestershire sauce

Salt and pepper to taste

Dredge the chicken in the rice flour. In a large soup pot, brown chicken in butter, add water, cover, and simmer over low heat for 20 minutes. Remove chicken from the pot; when cool enough to handle, take the meat from the bones. Discard bones.

While the chicken is cooling, stir the tomatoes, vegetables, cloves, and Worcestershire sauce into the pot and cook until tender, another 15 minutes.

Return the chicken meat to the pot and simmer for another 5 minutes. Season with salt and pepper. Serve with rice or mashed potatoes on the side.

A Flour You Can Love

Rice flour is a godsend for people who cannot tolerate gluten. This versatile and highly nutritious gluten-free flour is packed with protein, B-vitamins, iron, and fiber.

440 calories | 21 g fat | 22.8 g carbohydrate | 38.41 g protein | 286 mg sodium | 1.13 g fiber

Recipes for 10-Day Gluten Detox

Panna Cotta

Yield: 6

INGREDIENTS

2 teaspoons water

2 teaspoons unflavored gelatin

1 cup whipping cream

⅓ cup sugar, or to taste

2 cups yogurt, cream, milk, or low-fat buttermilk, well shaken

1 teaspoon vanilla

Fruit coulis or fresh fruit of your choice

Why Yogurt is Your Friend

Rich in calcium, protein, iron, and vitamins A and C, yogurt helps cleanse the intestinal tract and also improves the bioavailability of other nutrients in the body.

Mix the water and gelatin together and let rest until gelatin "blooms," about 5 minutes.

Stir the cream and sugar in a saucepan over moderate heat until sugar dissolves. Do not boil. Whisk in the gelatin and water; cool to room temperature. Whisk in yogurt and vanilla.

Prepare six 6-ounce custard cups with nonstick spray. Divide the custard between the cups. Refrigerate for 6 hours or overnight.

Run a sharp knife around the edge of each cup. Invert the cups on chilled plates. Serve with fruit coulis or fresh berries or both.

223 calories | 15.4 g fat | 16.2 g carbohydrate | 4.8 g protein | 102 mg sodium | 0 g fiber

Wild Rice Salad

Serves: 6

INGREDIENTS

4 cups water

¾ cup uncooked wild rice

1 teaspoon salt and black pepper to taste

1 small red onion, chopped

3 stalks celery, finely chopped

1 cup water chestnuts, drained and chopped

1 cup jicama, peeled and chopped

⅔ cup olive oil

⅓ cup raspberry vinegar

½ cup fresh Italian flat-leaf parsley, chopped

6 ounces fresh raspberries, rinsed and set on paper towels to dry

Bring water to boil and add the rice; return to a rolling boil and then reduce heat to simmer and cover tightly. After 30 minutes, add salt and pepper.

When the rice has bloomed but is still hot, add the vegetables and apple. Taste and add salt and pepper.

Mix the olive oil and vinegar together with the parsley and combine the rice and vegetables. Place in a large serving dish and serve warm or chilled. Sprinkle with berries at the last minute.

351 calories | 24.53 g fat | 28.42 g carbohydrate | 4 g protein | 395 mg sodium | 2 g fiber

Wild about Wild Rice

Forget about Minute Rice! Wild rice has three times the fiber; twice the protein, vitamin B6, and iron; four times the vitamin E; and ten times the folic acid of white rice, as well as vitamin K, thiamin, and riboflavin, which aren't found in white rice at all. Because people with gluten intolerance are often lacking in folic acid as well as vitamins B6, E, and K, wild rice is a delicious way to close nutritional gaps.

Recipes for 10-Day Gluten Detox

Beef Stroganoff

Serves: 6

INGREDIENTS

2 tablespoons olive oil

4 shallots, peeled and chopped

8 ounces tiny button mushrooms, brushed clean, stems removed

2 garlic cloves, minced

2 tablespoons tapioca flour plus ¼ cup for coating the meat

1 teaspoon dried mustard

Salt and pepper to taste

1½ cups beef broth, warmed

1 cup dry red wine

1 teaspoon gluten-free Worcestershire sauce

2 pounds filet mignon, cut into bite-size cubes

2 tablespoons unsalted butter

2 tablespoons snipped fresh dill weed

1 cup sour cream or crème frâiche

In a large sauté pan, heat the oil over medium heat and add the shallots, mushrooms, and garlic. Cook for 5 minutes to soften. Add the flour, mustard, and salt and pepper, stirring to blend.

Mix in the warmed beef broth, cook and stir to thicken. Stir in the wine and Worcestershire sauce and bring to a boil. Turn off the heat.

On a large piece of waxed paper, roll the beef in flour. Heat the unsalted butter in a separate pan. Sear the beef in the butter. Spoon the beef into the mushroom sauce, add the dill weed and sour cream, and stir to blend. Simmer for 10 to 15 minutes; the beef should be medium rare.

---

436 calories | 28.8 g fat | 8.5 g carbohydrate | 35.37 g protein | 292 mg sodium | .48 g fiber

Recipes for 10-Day Gluten Detox

Grilled Eggplant Parmesan

Serves: 2

INGREDIENTS

1 large eggplant, sliced into ½-inch slices

2 tablespoons extra-virgin olive oil, divided

Salt and pepper to taste

1 small white onion, diced

2 teaspoons garlic, minced

4 large Roma tomatoes, seeded and chopped

1 tablespoon sugar

1½ teaspoons Italian parsley, minced

½ cup grated Parmesan cheese

¼ cup grated mozzarella cheese

Why Eggplant is So Accommodating

Rich in B vitamins and niacin, calcium, and potassium, eggplant has a bland flavor that blends in well with other ingredients. It helps cleanse and soothe the bladder and kidneys.

Brush eggplant with 1 tablespoon olive oil. Season with kosher salt and pepper. Grill on hot well-oiled grill for 1–2 minutes per side, just until eggplant begins to brown and soften.

Sauté onion in 1 tablespoon olive oil until soft. Add garlic and sauté 30 seconds. Add tomatoes and sugar. Simmer for 20 minutes.

Place eggplant in baking dish coated with cooking spray. Top each slice of eggplant with tomato sauce. Sprinkle cheeses on top.

Bake in a 350°F oven covered with foil for 20 minutes.

Uncover and bake for 5 minutes or until cheese is bubbly.

450 calories | 23.9 g fat | 39.11 g carbohydrate | 19.4 g protein | 568 mg sodium | 4.2 g fiber

Stuffed Pork Chops

Serves: 4

INGREDIENTS

1 tart apple, peeled, cored and chopped

½ cup chopped onion

1 tablespoon dried rosemary, crumbled, or 2 tablespoons chopped fresh

¼ cup finely chopped Italian flat leaf parsley

½ cup olive oil

½ cup gluten-free cornbread crumbs

Salt and pepper to taste

4 thick-cut pork rib chops

¼ cup olive oil

4 garlic cloves, chopped

2 medium onions, chopped

½ cup chicken broth

½ cup dry white wine

Zest and juice of ½ lemon

2 ripe pears, peeled, cored and quartered

2 teaspoons cornstarch mixed with 2 ounces cold water (to thicken the gravy)

Sauté the apple, onion, and herbs in ½ cup olive oil. When softened, add the cornbread crumbs, salt, and pepper. When cool enough to handle, stuff into the chops and secure with toothpicks.

Add ¼ cup olive oil to the pan and brown the chops on medium high. Add the rest of the ingredients, except for the cornstarch-and-water mixture, and cover. Simmer for 40 minutes over very low heat.

Place the chops on a warm platter and add the cornstarch-and-water mixture to the gravy in the pan if you want it to be thicker. Add salt and pepper to taste.

---

763 calories | 49 g fat | 40 g carbohydrate | 32 g protein | 745 mg sodium | 3 g fiber

The Magic of Pears

Like all fruits, pears are gluten free. Rich in fiber as well as vitamins C, B, folic acid, niacin, and the minerals phosphorous and calcium, pears help reduce disorders of the bladder, liver, and prostate, and also help relieve constipation.

Chapter 6

10-Day Lactose Detox

YOU'RE AT YOUR LOCAL STARBUCKS polishing off your second latte when you suddenly feel queasy. Could you be lactose intolerant—at your age? The answer is yes. Lactose intolerance is the inability to digest lactose, a sugar found in milk products. This condition affects millions of American adults. The 10-Day Lactose Detox plan will help you determine if you may be lactose intolerant. Although not serious, once you develop lactose intolerance, it's necessary to reduce or eliminate your consumption of milk products to avoid symptoms.

Understanding Lactose Intolerance

Lactose intolerance is caused when the small intestine fails to make a sufficient amount of the enzyme, lactase, which the body needs to digest the milk sugar, lactose.

According to the National Digestive Diseases Information Clearinghouse (NDDIC), there are two types of lactose intolerance: primary and secondary lactase deficiency. The primary version develops over several years as the body gradually makes less lactase. Secondary lactase deficiency is caused by injuries to the small intestines that may be caused by a variety of factors, including celiac disease, Crohn's disease, chemotherapy, and diseases accompanied by severe diarrhea.

According to the NDDIC, lactose deficiency may be genetic. Scientists are currently developing tests that may help people determine their risk for developing lactose intolerance if one or both parents have the condition.

If you have lactose intolerance, you may start feeling symptoms anywhere from 30 minutes to 2 hours after consuming a milk product. Symptoms include:

- Bloating
- Cramps
- Flatulence
- Heartburn

- Nausea
- Constipation
- Diarrhea
- Foul-smelling stools
- Malnutrition
- Weight loss
- Headache
- Fatigue

Because symptoms of lactose intolerance mimic many other digestive problems and diseases, it may be difficult for your physician to diagnose your condition solely on symptoms. If your physician suspects you suffer from lactose intolerance, he may have you eliminate all milk products for a week to see if your symptoms improve, or use one of several tests to diagnose the condition.

> **Food for Thought**
> *If you have severe lactose intolerance, you may also want to check all the ingredients in your medications to ensure they don't contain lactose, which is sometimes found in birth control pills and over-the-counter products like antacids.*

Treating Lactose Intolerance

The easiest and fastest way to "cure" lactose intolerance is to avoid or reduce your intake of milk products that cause symptoms. Studies show that most people with lactose intolerance may be able to tolerate a small amount of lactose without developing symptoms, or anywhere from 2–4 ounces of milk product. Some people with lactose intolerance find that using dietary lactase enzyme supplements, such as Lactaid, allows them to continue to enjoy dairy products. They are available over the counter.

If you're lactose intolerant, you may want to try small amounts of the following milk products before crossing them off your list:

- Buttermilk
- Goat's milk
- Yogurt and other fermented milk products
- Ice cream and milkshakes
- Hard or aged cheeses

Sleuthing Out Lactose

Many processed foods contain small amounts of "hidden" milk products to extend their shelf life. These foods include:

- Bread, crepes, cookies, biscuits, scones, rolls, cakes, pie crust, and prepared baking mixes
- Processed breakfast foods, including cereals, doughnuts, frozen waffles and pancakes, toaster pastries, and sweet rolls
- Instant soups and potatoes
- Breakfast drinks and liquid and powdered milk-based meal replacements
- Processed snacks, including potato chips, corn chips
- Processed meats, including hot dogs, lunch meat, bacon, and sausage
- Margarine
- Store-bought salad dressings
- Protein powders and bars
- Candy
- Nondairy liquid and powdered coffee creamers
- Nondairy whipped toppings

Meal Plans for 10-Day Lactose Detox

As you begin to eliminate lactose from your diet, you will likely find you have more energy, fewer headaches, weight gain, and/or sinus problems! The benefits largely outweigh the negatives when it comes to abandoning dairy, which should make it easier for you to commit to this kind of lifestyle change.

Day 1

Breakfast
1 cup Banana-Raspberry Smoothie (page 91)
1 Hardboiled Egg
1 slice Toasted French Bread
Herbal Tea or Coffee

Lunch
1½ cups Chicken and Vegetable Stir-Fry
¾ cup Noodles
Iced Herbal Tea

Dinner
1 cup Sirloin Tips with Mushrooms and Garlic
¾ Brown Rice
1 cup Steamed Broccoli and Carrots
½ cup Apple Crisp
Herbal Tea

Day 2

Breakfast
1 Veggie Phyllo Breakfast Pocket
½ cup Melon with Berries
8 ounces Soy Milk
Herbal Tea or Coffee

Lunch
2 (4-inch) slices Basil Bruschetta with Portobello and Feta
½ cup Seedless Watermelon and Grapes
Herbal Tea

Dinner
4 ounces Grilled Citrus Mahi Mahi (page 92)
½ cup Sautéed Spinach
½ cup Roasted New Potatoes
½ cup Mango Sorbet
Herbal Tea

Day 3

Breakfast
1 cup Soy Yogurt with Strawberries, Raisins, and Walnuts
1 slice Toasted Italian Bread
Herbal Tea

Lunch
1 Smoked-Turkey Bagel Sandwich
1 cup Vegetable Soup
Herbal Tea

Dinner
1 serving Ginger Beef Stir-Fry (page 93)
1 cup White Rice
½ cup Steamed Asparagus
1 cup Green Salad
1 slice Angel Food Cake with Sliced Peaches
Herbal Tea

Meal Plans for 10-Day Lactose Detox

Breakfast

¾ cup Steel-Cut Oatmeal
    with Cinnamon and Raisins
1 slice Canadian Bacon
6 ounces Fresh Orange Juice
Herbal Tea

Lunch

1 serving Thai Chicken Salad
    (page 94)
10 Wheat-Thin-Style
    Crackers
Herbal Tea

Dinner

4 ounces Broiled Lamb Chop
1 cup Garlic Couscous
½ cup Minted Peas
1 cup Gelatin Dessert with
    Mixed Fruit
Herbal Tea

Breakfast

1 serving Scrambled Eggs
    (page 95)
½ cup Cooked Corn Grits
½ Grapefruit
Herbal Tea

Lunch

2 cups Ground Beef Taco
    Salad with Soy Cheese
½ cup Baked Corn Tortilla
    Chips with Salsa
Herbal Tea

Dinner

4 ounces Roasted Garlic
    Chicken
½ cup Noodles with Dairy-
    Free Margarine
1 cup Steamed Green Beans
    with Lemon
½ cup Grilled Peaches with
    Frozen Vanilla Soy Dessert
Herbal Tea

Breakfast

½ cup Muesli with Soy Milk
    and Chopped Dates
1 sliced Apple with Peanut
    Butter
Herbal Tea

Lunch

1 Tuna Salad Sandwich on a
    French Baguette
1 cup Minestrone Soup
Herbal Tea

Dinner

1 Grilled Pork Chops with
    Pineapple Salsa (page 96)
1 cup Sautéed Swiss Chard
1 small Baked Sweet Potato
½ cup Raspberry Sorbet with
    Berries
Herbal Tea

Breakfast

1 cup Cream of Wheat
    Cereal (not instant)
1 cup Soy Milk
½ cup Melon Slices with
    Blueberries
Herbal Tea

Lunch

1½ cups Manhattan Clam
    Chowder
¼ cup Oyster Crackers
½ cup Fennel and Pink
    Grapefruit Salad
Herbal Tea

Dinner

¾ cup Green Chili Chicken
    (page 97)
1 cup White Rice
1 cup Green Salad
1 Frozen Strawberry Fruit Bar
Herbal Tea

Meal Plans for 10-Day Lactose Detox

Day 8

Breakfast
1 Rice Cake with Peanut Butter and Jam
1 cup Soy Milk
1 sliced Orange
Herbal Tea

Lunch
4 ounces Teriyaki-Glazed Chicken
½ cup Brown Rice
1 serving Asian-Style Coleslaw (page 98)
Herbal Tea

Dinner
6 ounces Barbecue Ribs
½ cup German Potato Salad
1 cup Sliced Tomatoes and Cucumbers
1 Baked Apple with Cinnamon and Nutmeg
Herbal Tea

Day 9

Breakfast
2 Scrambled Eggs with Spinach, Mushrooms, and Diced Tomato
1 slice Toasted Italian Bread
½ cup Mixed Fruit Salad
Herbal Tea

Lunch
1 cup Vegetarian Chili with Soy Cheddar Cheese
¼ cup Corn Tortilla Chips
1 cup Green Salad
Herbal Tea

Dinner
4-ounce Marinated Flank Steak (page 99)
1 medium-size Baked Potato
1 cup Summer Squash Sauté
1 Grilled Pear with Vanilla Frozen Soy Dessert
Herbal Tea

Day 10

Breakfast
1 Banana Muffin (made with soy milk)
2 ounces Canadian Bacon
½ cup Strawberries and Blackberries
Herbal Tea

Lunch
2 cups Pasta and Vegetable Salad with 3 ounces Grilled Shrimp
Herbal Tea

Dinner
1¼ cups Chicken Fajitas with Bell Pepper and Onions
2 Corn Tortillas
½ cup Mexican Rice
1 cup Green Salad
1 Banana Orange Cupcake (page 100)
Herbal Tea

Part II: Elimination Detox Diets

Banana Raspberry Smoothie

Serves: 4

INGREDIENTS

2 cups frozen raspberries

2 bananas, sliced

1 cup rice milk

1 cup frozen dairy-free Tofutti frozen dessert

½ teaspoon cinnamon

⅛ teaspoon cardamom

Combine all ingredients in blender or food processor. Blend or process until mixture is smooth. Serve immediately.

278.30 calories | 2.82 g fat | 61.92 g carbohydrate | 3.16 g protein | 58.40 mg sodium | 3.36 g fiber

The Queen of Berries

Rich in antioxidants vitamin C and manganese, raspberries helps fight free-radical damage to cells. Studies show the anthocyanins in raspberries reduce the risk of heart disease, and delay the effects of aging. Raspberries also contain quercetin, an antioxidant that reduces allergic reactions, inflammation, and pain.

Recipes for 10-Day Lactose Detox

Grilled Citrus Mahi Mahi

Serves: 2

INGREDIENTS

½ cup fresh orange juice

½ cup pink grapefruit juice

¼ cup fresh lime juice

1 teaspoon lime zest

½ cup dry sherry

2 tablespoons fresh grated gingerroot

¼ cup low-sodium soy sauce

1 tablespoon sesame oil

½ teaspoon salt and pepper

2 teaspoons chili powder

2–8 ounces Mahi Mahi fillets, rinsed

Combine citrus juices, zest, sherry, soy sauce, ginger, sesame oil, salt and pepper, and chili powder. Pour over fish and marinate in refrigerator for 2 hours.

Grill fish on well-oiled grill.

Discard marinade.

438 calories | 14.66 g fat | 20.81 g carbohydrate | 39.55 g protein | 1,676 mg sodium | .69 g fiber

A True Fish Story

The essential fatty acids in Mahi Mahi help build strong cell membranes, prevent degenerative diseases, reduce the incidence of asthma, and provide a steady source of energy.

Ginger Beef Stir-Fry

Serves: 2

INGREDIENTS

6 ounces top sirloin, fat trimmed

2 large green onions, finely chopped

2 tablespoons gingerroot, finely grated

4 tablespoons low-sodium soy sauce

2 tablespoons dark brown sugar

2 tablespoons sesame oil

2 large garlic cloves, minced

⅛ teaspoon black pepper

¼ cup peanut oil (for frying)

½ cup pea pods, sliced

Open Sesame

Sesame oil, a plant-based oil high in essential fatty acids, lends a nutty, sweet flavor to dishes and also offers a host of health benefits, including lowering cholesterol and blood pressure, reducing stress, and relaxing aching muscles.

Slice beef into stir–fry-style strips.

Mix green onion, gingerroot, soy sauce, brown sugar, sesame oil, garlic, and pepper to form meat marinade. Marinate meat for at least 2 hours in the refrigerator. Return to room temperature prior to cooking.

Heat a wok or large sauté pan and add peanut oil. Stir-fry beef strips. Remove beef and set aside.

Add additional peanut oil if necessary and cook pea pods until light brown and crisp. Return beef to pan and cook on high heat until heated through.

Serve immediately.

496 calories | 37 g fat, 6.94 g saturated fat | 15.82 g carbohydrate | 24.57 g protein | 967mg sodium | 1.1 g fiber

Thai Chicken Salad

Serves: 4

INGREDIENTS

20 ounces boneless, skinless, organic chicken breast

3 tablespoons low-sodium soy sauce, divided

2 garlic cloves, minced

1 teaspoon hot pepper flakes (optional)

6 tablespoons fresh lime juice

¼ cup light brown sugar

1 serrano green chili, minced

1 tablespoon fresh gingerroot, peeled and minced

1 tablespoon minced cilantro

3 cups romaine lettuce, chopped

1 yellow bell pepper, cut into strips

1 red bell pepper, cut into strips

½ cucumber, peeled and chopped

Marinate chicken in 1 tablespoon soy sauce, 1 minced garlic clove, and red pepper flakes. Marinate for at least 30 minutes and up to 24 hours.

To make dressing whisk together the lime juice, 2 tablespoons soy sauce, 1 minced garlic clove, brown sugar, serrano chili, gingerroot, and cilantro.

Remove chicken from marinade. Discard marinade. Grill chicken and cut into strips.

Toss lettuce with dressing. Place on chilled plate with chicken, bell pepper, and cucumber.

260 calories | 4.3 g fat | 16.94 g carbohydrate | 38.15 g protein | 572 mg sodium | 1 g fiber

Cilantro Ole!

This herb is often found in Mexican cuisine and is said to be an acquired taste. Because cilantro is renowned for its anticholesterol, antidiabetic, and anti-inflammatory effects, it's well worth cultivating a taste for.

Scrambled Eggs

Serves: 4

INGREDIENTS

2 tablespoons olive oil

8 eggs

2 tablespoons water

½ teaspoon salt

Dash white pepper

Heat medium skillet over medium heat. Add olive oil. Meanwhile, combine remaining ingredients in a medium bowl and beat until frothy.

Add egg mixture to pan and cook, running a heatproof spatula along the bottom occasionally, until eggs form soft curds that are just set. Serve immediately.

206.67 calories | 16.69 g fat | .77 g carbohydrate | 12.49 g protein | 430.82 mg sodium | 0 g fiber

The Incredible Edible Egg

Once blamed for high cholesterol, eggs are now considered a healthy and safe way to meet protein needs, according to the American Heart Association. Research conducted at Harvard University showed that eating eggs daily did not increase the cholesterol levels of people with healthy cholesterol levels.

Recipes for 10-Day Lactose Detox

Grilled Pork Chops with Pineapple Salsa

Serves: 4

INGREDIENTS

1 tablespoon extra-virgin olive oil

3 teaspoons cumin

1 teaspoon garlic powder

½ teaspoon kosher salt and black pepper

4 boneless pork chops, trimmed of fat

½ cup red onion, finely diced

1 teaspoon lime zest

Juice of 1 lime

½ large pineapple, peeled and diced

Stir olive oil, cumin, garlic, salt, and pepper in a small bowl.

Rub olive oil mixture on pork chops.

Make salsa with onion, lime juice and zest, and pineapple.

Grill pork chops on hot, well-oiled grill. Serve with salsa.

377 calories | 12.48 g fat | 35.54 g. carbohydrate | 30.7 g protein | 1,068 mg sodium | 1.97 g fiber

Pineapple Power

High in vitamins C and A, calcium, and potassium, pineapples contain bromelain, an enzyme that facilitates digestion, helps decrease inflammation, and relaxes smooth muscles.

Recipes for 10-Day Lactose Detox

Green Chili Chicken

Serves: 6

INGREDIENTS

6 boneless, skinless chicken breasts

1 (4-ounce) can chopped green chilies, drained

1 cup frozen corn

2 tomatoes, chopped

2 tablespoons fresh lime juice

¼ cup chopped cilantro

½ teaspoon salt

⅛ teaspoon cayenne pepper

1 teaspoon cumin

Hot Chilies for Weight Loss

Green chilies are a potent antioxidant, containing more vitamin C, ounce for ounce, than any citrus fruit. In addition, studies show that green chilies are a boon for dieters. They result in a tenfold increase in weight loss by reducing cravings for sweet and fatty foods.

Preheat oven to 375°F. Cut six 12-inch squares of parchment paper and place on work surface. Place a chicken breast in center of each.

In medium bowl, combine chilies, corn, tomatoes, lime juice, cilantro, salt, pepper, and cumin, and mix well. Divide on top of chicken.

Fold edges of parchment paper over chicken and crimp to close. Place on cookie sheet and bake until chicken is cooked and parchment paper is browned, about 25–35 minutes. Serve immediately.

182.28 calories | 3.43 g fat | 9.48 g carbohydrate | 43 g protein | 483.29 mg sodium | 1 g fiber

Recipes for 10-Day Lactose Detox

Asian-Style Coleslaw

Serves: 2

INGREDIENTS

¼ cup Smart Beat mayonnaise

1 tablespoon mirin

1 tablespoon unseasoned rice vinegar

½ tablespoon, low-sodium soy sauce

½ tablespoon apple cider vinegar

1 cup red cabbage, finely shredded

1 cup napa cabbage, finely shredded

½ cup carrot, peeled and julienned

½ small seedless cucumber, peeled and thinly sliced

2 green onions, thinly sliced

½ teaspoon salt and pepper, to taste

In a large bowl, combine the mayonnaise, mirin, rice vinegar, soy sauce, and apple cider vinegar to make dressing.

Place cabbage, carrot, cucumber, and green onion in large bowl and toss with dressing. Taste and add salt and pepper if needed.

Refrigerate.

43 calories | .22 g fat | 8.5 g carbohydrate | 1.86 g protein | 697 mg sodium | 1.31 g fiber

The King of Cruciferous

Cabbage contains a host of phytochemicals, vitamins, minerals, and fiber that are important to your health. Studies show that sulforaphane—one of the phytochemicals found in cabbage—stimulates enzymes in the body that detoxify carcinogens before they damage cells.

Marinated Flank Steak

Serves: 4

INGREDIENTS

⅓ cup dry red wine

2 tablespoons brown sugar

1 tablespoon honey

2 tablespoons beef stock

2 cloves garlic, minced

1 onion, minced

1 jalapeño pepper, minced (optional)

⅛ teaspoon black pepper

½ teaspoon salt

1½ pounds flank steak

How Do You Cut Flank Steak?

Flank steak has a clearly defined grain running through the meat. This looks like fine lines in the flesh. When you cut flank steak, whether you're cutting it before cooking or after, it must be cut against the grain. That means you should make your cuts perpendicular to the lines in the meat.

In a large ziplock food-storage bag, combine all ingredients except flank steak. Add steak, seal bag, and knead bag gently to mix.

Place bag in large pan and refrigerate 18–24 hours, turning bag occasionally.

When ready to eat, prepare and heat grill. Remove steak from marinade; discard marinade.

Grill steak 6 inches from medium coals 12–16 minutes, turning once, until desired doneness. Cover and let stand 5 minutes. Slice across grain to serve.

302.20 calories | 11.55 g fat | 1.50 g carbohydrate | 35 g protein | 135.92 mg sodium | 1g fiber

Banana Orange Cupcakes

Serves: 18

INGREDIENTS

1½ cups all-purpose flour

½ cup whole wheat flour

1½ teaspoons baking powder

½ teaspoon baking soda

½ teaspoon salt

¼ cup olive or vegetable oil

1 ripe banana, mashed

¾ cup rice milk

½ cup orange juice

¼ cup honey

2 teaspoons vanilla

2 teaspoons grated orange zest

1 cup powdered sugar

2 tablespoons orange juice

Orange-Aid

A rich source of vitamins C, B, and K; biotin; folic acid; amino acids; and minerals, oranges cleanse the gastrointestinal track, strengthen capillary walls, and benefit the heart and lungs.

Preheat oven to 350°F. In large bowl, combine flours, baking powder, baking soda, and salt and mix well with wire whisk.

In medium bowl, combine oil, banana, and rice milk and mash together using a potato masher. Stir in ½ cup orange juice, honey, vanilla, and orange zest and mix well.

Add banana mixture all at once to the dry ingredients and mix until combined. Stir 1 minute.

Fill prepared cups ¾ full. Bake 18–23 minutes or until cupcakes are set and light golden brown. Let cool on wire rack 10 minutes.

In small bowl, combine powdered sugar and 2 tablespoons orange juice and mix well. Drizzle over warm cupcakes. Let cool completely.

131.39 calories | 3.42 g fat | 24.13 g carbohydrate | 1.96 g protein | 111.67 mg sodium | .17 g fiber

Chapter 7

5-Day Acid Balance Detox

IF YOUR BLOOD IS TOO ACIDIC, a condition called acidosis may be forcing your body to rob essential minerals like sodium, potassium, and calcium from your bones and organs to buffer the excess acid and remove it from the body. While most healthy people have a sufficient amount of alkaline reserves for everyday purposes, when acidic overload becomes chronic, it depletes the body's alkaline reserves. The most common cause of acidosis is consuming a diet that's too high in acid-producing foods, although chronic stress, excessive exercise, immune reactions, and heavy metal toxins may also deplete alkaline reserves. The 5-Day Acid Balance revolves around alkaline-producing foods that help restore your body's healthy acid/alkaline balance.

The Importance of Acid-Alkaline Balance

When your blood becomes overly acidic, it creates an environment in your body in which disease and illness can easily thrive. If your diet doesn't contain enough minerals to compensate for excess acidity, it decreases the cell's ability to produce energy and repair damaged cells. The result is illness, fatigue, and premature aging caused by acid waste.

A food is classified as either acidic or alkaline based on the effect the food has on urine pH. If a food increases the acid pH of urine after being eaten, it is generally considered an acid-producing food. If the food increases the urine's alkalinity after being ingested, it is considered an alkaline-producing food. The effect foods have on urine pH may be quite different than the actual pH level of foods. For instance, although citrus fruit is highly acidic, when ingested, it causes the urine to become alkaline.

Maintaining a Healthy pH

Your blood must stay within a small margin of pH, as even a slight deviation will cause your organs, lungs, skin, and digestive system to work harder to maintain a proper acid/alkaline balance. The ideal pH of your blood to fight off disease and infection is 7.36. If your blood acid levels become too high, acidosis occurs, providing a fertile environment for microorganisms to thrive. If your blood acidity level falls by just .36 percent, or to 7.0, you could go into a coma and die.

Maintaining a healthy blood pH has a variety of health benefits, including:

- Maintaining normal body weight
- Preventing obesity and overweight
- Maintaining a proper balance of insulin
- Moderating cholesterol levels
- Regulating blood pressure
- Moderating electrolyte balance in the body, which in turn promotes a healthy heart
- Preventing premature aging
- Maintaining healthy bones, teeth, and cartilage
- Boosting the immune system
- Promoting healthy digestion and elimination

> **Food for Thought**
>
> *According to the Mayo Clinic, imbalances in your blood pH can lead to a variety of health problems ranging from constipation, digestive problems, and headaches to heartburn, colds, fatigue, insomnia, muscle aches and pains, and itching. Some experts believe that diets high in acid-producing foods may trigger insulin sensitivity and lead to diabetes, the early formation of cancer, heart disease, diabetes, and Alzheimer's disease.*

Dietary Interventions to Acidosis

The Standard American Diet, or SAD, is partially to blame for acidosis because it contains high amounts of animal products (meat, eggs, and dairy) that are high in acid-producing substances, and low in alkaline-producing substances. Other acid-producing foods that are staples of the SAD include white flour, sugar, coffee, and soft drinks.

One of the best ways to maintain a healthy balance of acid- and alkaline-producing foods in the body is to consume a diet comprised of 60 percent alkaline-forming foods, and 40 percent acid-forming foods. But if your acid level is too high, you can reduce levels safely by consuming a diet made up of 80 percent alkaline-producing foods, and 20 percent acid-producing foods.

Acid-Producing Foods

The most common acid-producing foods in the American diet include grain products, white sugar, lentils, olives, beans, oils, meat, animal fats, seafood, blueberries, canned or glazed fruits, cranberries, currants, plums, prunes, corn, winter squash, butter, cheese, tea, coffee, sour apples, cream, cocoa, sour grapes, soft drinks, flour products, wheat germ, distilled vinegar, and snack foods that are high in sugar and trans fat.

Other foods that are acid-producing include liver and other organ meats, gravy and broth, wine, beer, sour cream, aged cheeses, yogurt, distilled water, and buttermilk, including buttermilk pancakes and biscuits.

> **DETOX TIP**
>
> If you use artificial sweeteners and suffer from acidosis, consider switching to sugar or honey. All artificial sweeteners, including NutraSweet, Spoonful, Sweet 'N Low, Equal, Splenda, are acid-producing substances.

Many prescription and over-the-counter drugs are also acid-producing, including aspirin, hydrochloric acid supplements, digestive aids, cough and flu medications, and probiotics or "helpful bacteria" used to treat bladder infections, diarrhea, and irritable bowel syndrome. In addition, vitamin B supplements are also acid producing.

Herbicides, pesticides, fungicides, and other chemicals used in agriculture are extremely acidic as well as unsafe. To decrease your risk of chemical contamination from pesticides and decrease your level of acidity, buy organic produce.

Low-Acid or Alkaline-Producing Foods

In general, fruits, green vegetables, spices, herbs, seasonings, nuts, and seeds are healthy alkaline-forming foods. Alkaline-producing foods also include almonds, dates, parsley, potatoes, string beans, molasses, peas, coconut, sweet corn, melons, carrots, maple syrup, squash, figs, spinach, chard, bananas, beets, okra, sweet peppers, avocado, lettuces, cucumbers, cabbage, and other cruciferous vegetables.

Other low-acid foods include dried fruit, pears, papayas, sweet apples, raspberries, strawberries, prunes, and raisins.

Meal Plans for 5-Day Acid Balance Detox

Once you become familiar with low-acid foods, you'll easily be able to modify this plan to suit your specific taste. There are several inexpensive over-the-counter pH tests available so you can check your progress along the way.

Day 1

Breakfast
1 cup Tofu Scramble (page 22)
1 Banana Pancake, 5-inch
6 ounces Fresh Apple Juice
Herbal Tea or Coffee

Lunch
1 serving Stuffed Mushrooms (page 106)
1 cup Green Salad
Herbal Tea

Dinner
4 ounces Grilled Swordfish with Avocado Salsa (page 107)
1 medium-size Baked Potato
½ cup Sautéed Spinach
1 Grilled Pineapple and Apricot Skewer
Herbal Tea

Day 2

Breakfast
1 serving Carrot, Ginger, Banana Smoothie (page 108)
1 sliced Apple with Almond Butter
Herbal Tea or Coffee

Lunch
3 ounces Cold Salmon with Salad Greens
1 Pita Bread
1 Pear
Herbal Tea

Dinner
4 ounces Baked Chicken
1 cup Rosemary Couscous
1 cup Mixed Greens with Dandelion Greens and Goat Cheese (page 109)
¾ cup Strawberry Sorbet

Day 3

Breakfast
2 Scrambled Eggs
1 slice Whole Wheat Toast
½ cup Sliced Strawberries, Bananas, and Blueberries
Herbal Tea

Lunch
1 serving Spinach Salad, Berries, and Almonds (page 110)
1 cup Vegetable Soup
Herbal Tea

Dinner
4 ounces Jerk-Seasoned Grilled Shrimp
½ cup Steamed Broccolini
1 serving Corn and Fresh Tomato Sauté
1 serving Mixed Fruit Salad in Lime Syrup (page 111)
Herbal Tea

Meal Plans for 5-Day Acid Balance Detox

Breakfast

1 serving Hawaiian Banana
Bread (page 112)
½ cup Mixed Fruit
Herbal Tea

Lunch

1 cup Split Pea Soup
1 cup Green Salad with Balsamic Vinaigrette
Herbal Tea

Dinner

4 ounces Turkey Medallions
with Mushroom Sauce
¾ cup Rice Pilaf
1 serving Maple Glazed Carrots (page 113)
1 cup Baby Spring Greens
Salad
Herbal Tea

Breakfast

1 cup Oatmeal with Dates
and Nuts
1 cup Soy Milk
½ cup Dried Apricots
Herbal Tea

Lunch

1 Tuna Veggie Wrap
½ cup Baked Sweet Potato
Fries (page 113)
1 cup Garden Salad
Herbal Tea

Dinner

2 Black Bean Tacos
½ cup Sauteed Spin-
ach with Tomatoes and
Crushed Red Pepper
Flakes
1 cup Garden Salad
1 serving Banana Boats
with Chocolate and Fresh
Strawberry Sauce (page
114)
Herbal Tea

Recipes for 5-Day Acid Balance Detox

Stuffed Mushrooms

Serves: 4

INGREDIENTS

8 large stuffing mushrooms, brushed clean

½ cup seasoned bread crumbs

½ cup red onion, minced

¼ cup extra-virgin olive oil

Salt and pepper to taste

Onions Help Memory

Onions, like citrus fruit, are an alkalizing vegetable that helps lower the acid content of your body. Onions contain fisetin, a naturally occurring flavonoid that stimulates pathways that improve long-term memory. Red onions contain anthocyanin and quercetin, and are even better for memory than yellow and white onions.

Preheat oven to 350°F.

Remove stems from mushrooms and hollow out caps.

Finely chop half of the stems and discard others.

In a small bowl combine chopped stems, bread crumbs, onion, and olive oil until well blended. Taste and season with salt and pepper.

Spoon mixture into mushrooms and place on ungreased cookie sheet.

Bake for 10–12 minutes or until golden brown. Serve immediately.

---

187 calories | 14.29 g fat, 1.98 g saturated fat | 11.1 g carbohydrate | 2.68 g protein | 94 mg sodium | .44 g fiber

Recipes for 5-Day Acid Balance Detox

Grilled Swordfish with Avocado Salsa

Serves: 2

INGREDIENTS

12 ounces swordfish steaks

Salt and black pepper, to taste

1 tablespoon extra-virgin olive oil

Juice of 1 lime

3 tablespoons lime peel, grated

2 Roma tomatoes, seeded and diced

1 small avocado, diced

½ cup red onion, diced

Rinse fish. Sprinkle with salt and pepper. Marinate for 30 minutes to 1 hour in olive oil, lime juice, lime peel.

To prepare salsa combine tomatoes, avocado, red onion, salt, and pepper.

Grill fish on well-oiled grill for 4–5 minutes per side or until cooked through.

Top fish with salsa.

403 calories | 25 g fat | 14.6 g carbohydrate | 28.75 g protein | 119 mg sodium | 2.4 g fiber

Can I Really Eat Citrus Fruit on a Low-Acid Diet?

Citrus fruits, including lime, lemon, oranges, and grapefruit, are highly acidic before you eat them, but once you eat them and your body metabolizes them, they become alkaline. Citrus fruits are loaded with vitamin C and other disease-fighting antioxidants, so eat up!

Carrot Ginger Banana Smoothie

Serves: 1

INGREDIENTS

2 carrots

½-inch piece fresh gingerroot, peeled

1 banana, cut into chunks

4 ice cubes

½ cup plain low-fat yogurt

Juice carrots and ginger in juicer.

Add carrot ginger juice to blender with banana, ice cubes and yogurt.

Blend well.

256 calories | 2.5 g fat, 1.39 g saturated fat | 49.5 g carbohydrate | 8.64 g protein | 134 mg sodium | 2 g fiber

Bugs Was Right

Carrots are a low-acid food that protect DNA, battle cataracts, and offer protection against certain cancers. Carrots are also high in beta-carotene, a potent antioxidant that fights free-radical damage. Carrots are high in vitamins A, B, and C, as well as calcium, potassium, and sodium.

Recipes for 5-Day Acid Balance Detox

Mixed Greens with Dandelion Greens and Goat Cheese

Serves: 2

INGREDIENTS

¼ cup extra-virgin olive oil

3 tablespoons balsamic vinegar

Salt and pepper to taste

6 ounces mixed salad greens (arugula, romaine, butter, endive)

1 cup dandelion greens

1 ounce goat cheese, crumbled

Full of Greens

Besides being very alkaline and extremely filling, mixed salad greens are high in vitamin C, folic acid, potassium, fiber, and beta-carotene, the antioxidant that fights heart disease.

Make dressing by whisking olive oil into balsamic vinegar. Season with salt and pepper.

Toss mixed greens and salad greens with balsamic dressing.

Place on chilled plates and crumble goat cheese on top.

---

359 calories | 32.89 g fat, 7.1 g saturated fat | 8.88 g carbohydrate | 7.23 g protein | 102 mg sodium | .76 g fiber

Recipes for 5-Day Acid Balance Detox

Spinach Salad, Berries, and Almonds

Serves: 2

INGREDIENTS

8 ounces baby spinach, stems removed

¼ cup balsamic vinegar

¼ cup extra-virgin olive oil

¼ cup feta cheese, crumbled

4 large strawberries, sliced

1 pear, sliced

⅛ cup roasted almonds

Place spinach leaves in bowl.

Make dressing by combining balsamic vinegar and oil in a small bottle and shaking well.

Toss dressing on spinach leaves. Add feta.

Place spinach on cold plates and top with berries, pear, and almonds.

Staying Alive with Spinach

Spinach helps with mental alertness and reduces the risk of certain cancers, including cancer of the liver, ovaries, colon, and prostate. Spinach is also packed with vitamins A, B, C, and K.

328 calories | 23 g fat | 22.39 g carbohydrate | 7.7 g protein | 249 mg sodium | 2.8 g fiber

Recipes for 5-Day Acid Balance Detox

Mixed Fruit Salad in Lime Syrup

Serves: 4

INGREDIENTS

1 medium honeydew melon, peeled and cubed

1 medium cantaloupe melon, peeled and cubed

1 large papaya, peeled, seeded and cubed

1 cup water

1 cup granulated sugar

¼ cup fresh lime juice and zest of 1 fresh lime

1 teaspoon rum extract

Combine fruit in bowl.

Heat water and sugar over medium low heat until sugar is dissolved. Remove from heat and stir in lime juice, zest, and rum extract.

Cool.

Pour over fruit and refrigerate for several hours to allow flavors to infuse into the fruit.

343 calories | .63 g fat, .03 g saturated fat | 82 g carbohydrate | 2.32 g protein | 28 mg sodium | 1.87g fiber

Recipes for 5-Day Acid Balance Detox

Hawaiian Banana Bread

Serves: 12

INGREDIENTS

1 cup granulated sugar

1 cup Smart Balance margarine

6 medium bananas, mashed

8 large egg whites

2½ cups cake flour

1 teaspoon salt

1 teaspoon ground cinnamon

1 teaspoon ground ginger

2 teaspoons baking soda

Yes, We Have Some Bananas

Because bananas are extremely alkaline, they can help lower the acid content of your blood. They are also high in fiber, which helps prevent constipation and helps regulate a healthy balance of acids and alkaline in the body, and rich in potassium, an essential electrolyte that maintains a proper fluid balance in the body.

Cream the sugar, margarine, bananas, and egg whites. Beat well.

Stir together flour, salt, cinnamon, ginger, and baking soda. Add to banana mixture.

Do not over mix.

Place into 2 greased 8" × 4" loaf pans.

Bake 375°F for 45–50 minutes or until a toothpick tester comes out clean.

Carefully remove from pan and cool before slicing.

285 calories | 7.98 g fat | 48.27 g carbohydrate | 5.09 g protein | 544 mg sodium | .41 g fiber

Recipes for 5-Day Acid Balance Detox

Maple Glazed Carrots

Serves: 2

INGREDIENTS

4 large carrots, peeled and cut into ½-inch-thick rounds

3 tablespoons unsalted butter

½ cup water

2 tablespoons pure maple syrup

1 tablespoon dark brown sugar

Salt and pepper to taste

Sauté carrots in unsalted butter until light brown.

Add water, brown sugar, and maple syrup and simmer until carrots are fork tender and most of the liquid is reduced to form a glaze over the carrots.

Season with salt and pepper.

297 calories | 16.93 g fat | 34 g carbohydrate | 2 g protein | 68 mg sodium | 1.87 g fiber

Baked Sweet Potato Fries

Serves: 4

INGREDIENTS

2 large sweet potatoes, skin on, scrubbed and cut into sticks ½ inch thick

2 tablespoons extra-virgin olive oil

1 tablespoon light brown sugar

1 teaspoon garlic powder

½ teaspoon salt and pepper

The Powerful Sweet Potatoe

Sweet potatoes are also very alkaline, and a delicious way to rebalance your diet. Sweet potatoes are rich in vitamins A and C—potent antioxidants that help boost your immunity, and fight disease.

Preheat oven to 450°F. Toss potatoes with olive oil, brown sugar, and garlic.

Line a baking sheet with foil and spray with pan spray.

Bake 15 minutes, stir and continue to bake for 10–15 minutes or until browned.

Remove from oven and sprinkle with salt and pepper while hot.

176 calories | 6.8 g fat, .95 g saturated fat | 26.73 g carbohydrate | 1.8 g protein | 293 mg sodium | .92 g fiber

Recipes for 5-Day Acid Balance Detox

Banana Boats with Chocolate and Fresh Strawberry Sauce

Serves: 2

INGREDIENTS

2 large bananas

4 cups semisweet chocolate chips

¼ cup sugar

¼ cup water

1 cup fresh strawberries, diced small

Split banana open lengthwise without cutting it all the way through. Press chocolate chips into the slit in the banana.

Wrap in foil and bake in 300°F oven for 5–10 minutes.

Combine sugar and water over medium heat. Heat until sugar is melted. Cool and add strawberries.

Serve banana with warm strawberry sauce.

330 calories | 8.16 g fat, 4.44 g saturated fat | 62 g carbohydrate | 2 g protein | 2 mg sodium | 4.4 g fiber

Chapter 8

30-Day Heavy Metal Detox

ENVIRONMENTAL TOXINS HAVE POISONED THE AIR WE BREATHE, the water we drink and bathe in, and the foods we eat, and account for 80 to 90 percent of all cancers, according to the National Cancer Institute. Environmental pollution has become so widespread that traces of DDT, a pesticide that was banned decades ago in the United States, are still found today in the ice at the North Pole. The 30-Day Heavy Metal Detox revolves around nutrients that displace heavy metals in your organs, and help your body eliminate them.

What is Heavy Metal?

A heavy metal is any metallic substance that has a high density, or is at least five times as dense as water. Heavy metals such as arsenic, cadmium, nickel, mercury, and lead, are so toxic that ingesting even a tiny amount can be dangerous or fatal because the body can't degrade or destroy them. Some of the twenty-three known heavy metals, including selenium, copper, zinc, and manganese, are required by the body in microscopic amounts to maintain health, but become toxic at higher amounts.

When you inhale, absorb, or otherwise ingest a dangerous heavy metal, your body cannot release or flush it from your system because of its high density. As a result, the heavy metals accumulate in your tissues, immune system, brain, and kidneys, where they impair bodily functions and contribute to serious conditions.

Heavy metals hide in many everyday products, including face creams, shampoos, personal care products, and household cleaning products. Because heavy metals are also used in agricultural and food processing and packaging, they may wind up in your food.

> **DETOX TIP**
>
> Aluminum, although not technically a heavy metal, can also be toxic when consumed in high amounts. If you're using aluminum pans for cooking, consider replacing them with cast iron pots, which boost the iron content of foods and eliminate the risk of heavy metal toxins.

The Dangerous Eight

According to scientists, the following eight heavy metals are the most dangerous to the human body. Here's what they are, and where they are most commonly found:

1. **Mercury:** Found in amalgam silver fillings, some vaccines, thermometers, old paint, pesticides, some fish, fluorescent lights, fabric softener, cosmetics, felt, and some medications.
2. **Lead:** Found in old paint, auto exhaust fumes, some hair colorings, candle wicks, stained glass, tap water, batteries, some pottery glazes, bullets, insecticides, and pewter ware.
3. **Nickel:** Found in dental crowns, root canals, cigarette smoke, stainless steel appliances, batteries, inexpensive jewelry, and hydrogenated cooking oils.
4. **Cadmium:** Found in cigarettes, dentures and pink dyes used in them, welding and auto exhaust fumes, ceramic glazes, many art supplies, Teflon, plastic, and fungicides.
5. **Aluminum:** Found in baking powder, some cooking utensils, aluminum foil, antiperspirants, some medications, cosmetics, and acid rain.
6. **Copper:** Found in some cooking pots, pans, and utensils, plumbing, gold fillings and crowns, and insecticides.
7. **Arsenic:** Found in tobacco smoke, smog, pesticides, wood preservatives, and green pigment used in toys, carpets, chalk, and curtains.
8. **Platinum:** Found in some dental gold fillings, and auto exhaust fumes.

Although there are hundreds of symptoms, the following are among the most common:

Mental disorders, including depression, anxiety, forgetfulness, poor memory, and temper tantrums.

Circulatory disorders, including numbness, tingling in the hands and feet, twitching of facial and other muscles, leg cramps, joint pain, and rapid heartbeat.

Intestinal disorders, including frequent urination, heartburn, abdominal bloating, kidney and liver damage, constipation and diarrhea, and loss of appetite.

Skin disorders, including excessive itching.

Nervous disorders, including tinnitus.

Impaired immunity and autoimmune disorders, such as lupus.

Symptoms tend to be mild and become worse with repeated exposure to heavy metals. For instance, repeated exposure to mercury may lead to loss of appetite, muscle tremors, depression, anxiety, emotional instability, and insomnia.

How to Cleanse Your Body of Heavy Metals

Although you can't completely eliminate all heavy metals from your body, you can dramatically lower the amount by consuming a diet high in nutrients that bind to or displace heavy metals in your body through a process called chelation.

The following nutrients displace heavy metals from your body and help your body eliminate them before they cause problems. Here's what they are, and the best dietary sources.

Calcium: Displaces mercury and lead in the body. Good sources of calcium include kale, parsley, watercress, beet greens, broccoli, spinach, romaine lettuce, string beans, oranges, carrots, celery, almonds, sesame seeds, and beans.

Magnesium: When consumed with calcium, magnesium helps displace mercury and lead. Good sources include beets, spinach, parsley, chard, carrots, cauliflower, blackberries, broccoli, and carrots,

Vitamin C: Increasing your consumption of foods high in vitamin C displaces lead and mercury in the body. Good sources include citrus fruit, broccoli, kale, parsley, Brussels sprouts, watercress, cauliflower, cabbage, strawberries, spinach, turnips, mangoes, cantaloupes, asparagus, and papaya.

Chlorophyll: Found in abundance in dark leafy green vegetables, chlorophyll binds to heavy metals. Good sources include spinach, broccoli, chard, kale, and lettuce.

Lipoic acid: A potent antioxidant that is essential for healthy metabolism, lipoic acid is a fatty acid that binds to heavy metals in the body and helps clear mercury and lead from the system. It is found in red meat, spinach, broccoli, potatoes, yams, carrots, beets, and Brewer's yeast.

Soluble fiber: Found in large amounts in fruits, vegetables, whole grains, nuts, seeds, and beans, soluble fiber helps the body draw out lead. Good sources include fruits, vegetables, whole grains, nuts, and seeds. About 20 to 30 percent of your diet should come from soluble fiber.

Sulfur: Lead, mercury, and cadmium rob the body of sulfur, which is essential for building cartilage and connective tissue. To avoid deficiencies caused by heavy metals consume foods high in sulfur: egg yolks, kelp, kale, turnips, raspberries, onions, cabbage, and mustard.

Zinc: The mineral zinc is destroyed by lead toxicity. Zinc is essential for healthy metabolism and for fighting free radicals, which attack cells and cause disease, impaired immunity, and premature aging. In addition, zinc deficiencies can lead to fatigue and contribute to neuropsychiatric disorders such as ADHD, depression, and dyslexia. Good sources of zinc include pumpkin seeds, gingerroot, carrots, garlic, parsley, spinach, cabbage, lettuce, and cucumbers.

Meal Plans for 30-Day Heavy Metal Detox

Stick to all-organic foods to get the best results from this detox plan. To amp it up even more, keep a fresh supply of cilantro or cilantro pesto on hand and add it to as many of your meals as possible. This wonder herb is inexpensive and sweeps heavy metals from your body. For Days 15–30, go to Day 1 and repeat the sequence.

Day 1

Breakfast

1 cup Oatmeal with Cinnamon
1 cup Low-Fat Milk or Soy Milk
Fresh Berries with Dollop of Yogurt
Herbal Tea

Lunch

1 wedge Broccoli Quiche (page 124)
1 cup Mixed Spring Greens Salad with Lemon Vinaigrette
Herbal Tea

Dinner

1 cup Beef Stew
⅔ cup Brown Rice
½ cup Sautéed Swiss Chard
1 Baked Apple with Ginger and Cinnamon (page 125)
1 cup Low-Fat Milk or Soy Milk
Herbal Tea

Day 2

Breakfast

2 Scrambled Eggs with Mushrooms and Spinach
2 slices Whole Wheat Toast
½ cup Fresh Cantaloupe
1 cup Low-Fat Milk

Lunch

2 cups Dark Green Veggie Salad with Nuts, Beans, Seeds, Broccoli, Cauliflower, and Fresh Yogurt-Tahini Dressing
1 serving Whole-Grain Crackers
Herbal Tea

Dinner

4 ounces Chicken Marsala
1 cup Wild Rice Pilaf
½ cup Green Beans with Slivered Almonds
½ cup Steamed Carrots
Herbal Tea

Day 3

Breakfast

1 cup Muesli with Nuts and Fruit
1 cup Low-Fat Milk or Soy Milk
1 ounce Canadian Bacon

Lunch

1 cup Lentil Soup (page 126)
1 small Whole-Grain Baguette
1 cup Caesar Salad
1 sliced Orange
Herbal Tea

Dinner

4 ounces Meatloaf
1 small Baked Potato
1 cup Mixed Vegetables
1 slice Garlic Bread
½ cup Pineapple Sorbet
Herbal Tea

Meal Plans for 30-Day Heavy Metal Detox

Day 4

Breakfast
1 small Whole Wheat Bagel with Peanut Butter and Whole Fruit Preserves
1 cup Mixed Fresh Fruit
1 cup Low-Fat Milk or Soy Milk

Lunch
1 Cajun-Seasoned Chicken Wrap with Mixed Greens
1 cup Tomato Cucumber Salad
Herbal Tea

Dinner
4 ounces Broiled Salmon
1 cup Sautéed Broccoli Rabe with Garlic and Pepper Flakes
½ cup Mashed Sweet Potatoes
1 Whole-Grain Roll
½ cup Grilled Apricots with a Dollop of Crème Fraîche
Herbal Tea

Day 5

Breakfast
1 cup Yogurt
½ cup Mixed Berries
1 slice Whole Wheat Toast with Almond Butter
Herbal Tea

Lunch
1 Roast Beef Sandwich on Whole-Grain Bread
1 cup Broccoli Salad (page 127)
1 cup Low-Fat Milk or Soy Milk
1 Pear

Dinner
1½ cups Vegetable Stir-Fry with Tofu
1 cup Brown Rice
½ cup Asian Pickled Cucumber Salad
3-inch square Fresh Gingerbread with a Dollop of Light Whipped Cream
Herbal Tea

Day 6

Breakfast
2-egg Omelet with Bell Pepper, Canadian Bacon, Onion, and Low-Fat Cheese
1 slice Whole-Grain Toast
1 cup Sliced Peaches and Blackberries
Herbal Tea

Lunch
1½ cups Minestrone Soup (see page 60)
1 cup Spinach Salad with Mushrooms and Balsamic Vinaigrette
1 serving Whole-Grain Crackers
1 cup Low-Fat Milk or Soy Milk

Dinner
1 serving Turkey Meatballs and Baby Bok Choy (page 128)
1 cup Linguini
1 cup Mixed Spring Greens Salad
½ cup Raspberry Sorbet with Fresh Chopped Pineapple
Herbal Tea

Part II: Elimination Detox Diets

Meal Plans for 30-Day Heavy Metal Detox

Breakfast

¾ cup Granola and Low-Fat
   Milk or Soy Milk
1 sliced Apple with Peanut
   Butter
Herbal Tea

Lunch

1½ cups Shrimp Cocktail
   with 4 ounces Shrimp
6 Whole-Grain Crackers
1 cup Mexican Rice
Herbal Tea

Dinner

1 broiled Lamb Chop
1 cup Couscous with Peas
   and Red Bell Pepper
½ cup Grilled Asparagus
1 cup Mixed Green Salad
½ cup Warm Figs with Goat
   Cheese and Honey
Herbal Tea

Day 7

Breakfast

1 Egg and Low-Fat Cheese
   Burrito with Whole Wheat
   Tortilla and Salsa
1 cup Carrot Apple Juice

Lunch

1 serving Cauliflower Soup
   (page 129)
1 slice Toasted Pumpernickel
   Bread
½ cup Butter Lettuce Salad
   with Tomatoes, Cucum-
   bers, and Red Onion
Herbal Tea

Dinner

1 Turkey-Spinach Burger on
   a Whole-Grain Bun
½ cup Cabbage Slaw with
   Sesame Seeds
½ cup Baked Sweet Potato
   Fries
½ cup Frozen Yogurt Parfait
   with Fresh Cherries
Herbal Tea

Day 8

Breakfast

1 small Whole-Grain Waffle
   with Peanut Butter and
   Cinnamon
1 cup Mango-Strawberry
   Yogurt Smoothie
Herbal Tea

Lunch

2 cups Greek Salad with
   Feta Cheese, Olives, and
   Lemon-Garlic Vinaigrette
½ Pita Bread with Hummus
Herbal Tea

Dinner

2 Southwest Chicken and
   Spinach Enchiladas with
   Low-Fat Cheese
½ cup Jicama Sticks with
   Lime Juice and Chili
   Seasoning
½ cup Brown Rice with
   Cilantro
2-inch-square Plum Tart
Herbal Tea

Day 9

Meal Plans for 30-Day Heavy Metal Detox

Day 10

Breakfast
1 wedge Cherry Clafouti
1 small handful of Walnuts
1 cup Low-Fat Milk or Soy Milk

Lunch
1 cup Spaghetti with Chick Peas and Fresh Basil Pesto
½ cup Sautéed Red, Yellow, and Orange Bell Peppers
Herbal Tea

Dinner
½ Roasted Cornish Game Hen with Wild Rice Stuffing
1 cup Mixed Green Salad
1 serving Roasted Cauliflower (page 130)
½ cup Mango Chunks and Blackberries with Vanilla Frozen Yogurt
Herbal Tea

Day 11

Breakfast
½ Cinnamon Raisin Bagel with Almond Butter
1 medium Tangerine
1 cup Low-Fat Milk or Soy Milk

Lunch
1 serving Mandarin Chicken Salad (page 131)
1 cup Miso Soup
Herbal Tea

Dinner
3 ounces Pot Roast with 1 cup Potatoes and Carrots
½ cup Steamed Broccoli
1 cup Mixed Green Salad with Radishes
½ cup Blueberry Cobbler
Herbal Tea

Day 12

Breakfast
1 cup Sweet Potato Hash with a Poached Egg and Canadian Bacon
1 cup Honeydew Melon Slices
1 cup Low-Fat Milk or Soy Milk

Lunch
1 grilled Portobello Mushroom Sandwich with Low-Fat Cheese
1 cup Broccoli, Cauliflower, Carrots, and Red Bell Pepper Marinated in Balsamic Vinaigrette
Herbal Tea

Dinner
3 ounces Baked Mushroom Chicken
1 serving Candied Brussels Sprouts (page 132)
½ cup Mashed Potatoes
1 Cabbage and Green Apple Slaw
2 Whole Wheat Dinner Rolls
½ cup Strawberry Sorbet with Sliced Bananas
Herbal Tea

Meal Plans for 30-Day Heavy Metal Detox

Breakfast

1 cup Granola
1 cup Yogurt
½ cup Mixed Berries
1 small handful Almonds
Herbal Tea

Lunch

1½ cup Spaghetti Squash
  with Ground Turkey and
  Marinara Sauce
1 cup Fennel and Grapefruit
  Salad
Herbal Tea

Dinner

5 ounces Grilled Tilapia in
  Lemon Caper Sauce
½ cup Rice Pilaf
½ cup Boiled Red Potatoes
  with Parsley
2 Whole Wheat Dinner Rolls
½ cup Tapioca Pudding
  made with Orange Juice
  and Pineapple
Herbal Tea

Breakfast

1 cup Oatmeal with Raisins,
  Nuts, and Cinnamon
2 slices Turkey Bacon
1 cup Low-Fat Milk or Soy
  Milk
6 ounces Fresh Orange Juice

Lunch

½ Whole Wheat Pita Bread
  Stuffed with Hummus and
  Veggies
1 cup Roasted Eggplant and
  Zucchini Slices
Herbal Tea

Dinner

4-ounce Grilled Beef Ten-
  derloin with Garlic and
  Fresh Herbs
1 serving Swiss Chard (page
  133)
½ cup Glazed Carrots
½ cup Noodles
1 cup Mixed Green Salad
½ cup Apple Crisp
Herbal Tea

Breakfast

½ Broiled Whole Wheat
  English Muffin with Low-
  Fat Cheese and Diced Bell
  Pepper
1 cup Pineapple, Banana,
  Mango Smoothie
Herbal Tea

Lunch

2 cups Spinach Salad with
  Grilled Shrimp
1 small Whole Grain
  Baguette
Herbal Tea

Dinner

3-inch square Spinach
  Lasagna
½ cup Summer Squash
  Sauté
1 cup Mixed Green Salad
1 slice Garlic Bread
½ cup Grilled Pineapple with
  Vanilla Yogurt
Herbal Tea

Recipes for 30-Day Heavy Metal Detox

Broccoli Quiche

Serves: 4

INGREDIENTS

4 eggs

1 cup half-and-half

½ medium onion, diced

1 tablespoon extra-virgin olive oil

2 cups broccoli, chopped

½ cup shredded cheddar cheese

½ cup part-skim mozzarella cheese, shredded

Salt and pepper to taste

Eat Your Broccoli!

Broccoli is a power food that's packed with fiber that clean-sweeps the intestines, removing heavy metal pollutants with waste. It also contains disease-fighting antioxidants that help fight disease and cancer. Did we mention it's also high in vitamins B6, C, and E?

Mix eggs with a mixer until light and fluffy.

Add half-and-half.

Sauté onion in olive oil until very soft. Add broccoli and sauté until just crisp.

Spray a 9-inch glass pie pan with cooking spray.

Place sautéed onions and broccoli in bottom of pie plate.

Sprinkle cheese on top.

Pour egg mixture over and add salt and pepper.

Bake in 325°F oven for 30 minutes, or until quiche is just set in the middle and light brown.

---

315 calories | 22 g fat, 9.5 g saturated fat | 8.8 g carbohydrate | 20.1 g protein | 237 mg sodium | .15 g fiber

Recipes for 30-Day Heavy Metal Detox

Baked Apple with Ginger and Cinnamon

Serves: 2

INGREDIENTS

2 golden delicious apples, cored
2 tablespoons unsalted butter
¼ cup dark brown sugar
2 teaspoons ground cinnamon
1 teaspoon ground ginger

An Apple a Day

Apples contain pectin, a fiber that absorbs toxins, stimulates digestion, and helps reduce cholesterol.

Spray baking dish with pan spray. Place apples in dish standing up.

In small saucepan melt butter. Add brown sugar, cinnamon, and ginger. Stir until sugar has dissolved.

Pour hot syrup into each apple. Pour extra syrup in baking dish.

Cover dish with foil.

Bake apples in 425°F oven until apples are tender; approximately 20–25 minutes.

296 calories | 11.85 g fat, 7 g saturated fat | 46.69 g carbohydrate | .58 g protein | 7 mg sodium | 4.53 g fiber

Recipes for 30-Day Heavy Metal Detox

Lentil Soup

Serves: 4

INGREDIENTS

2 large cloves garlic, minced

1 cup celery, diced

1 large onion, diced

3 tablespoons extra-virgin olive oil

1 cup dried lentils

2 large bay leaves

1 teaspoon cumin

1 teaspoon dried thyme

1 cup water

1 cup low-sodium chicken broth

1 cup canned tomatoes, diced

Salt and pepper to taste

Sauté the garlic, celery, and onion in olive oil.

Add remaining ingredients and simmer until tender.

Add salt and pepper to taste.

Ladle into warm soup bowls.

---

349 calories | 12 g fat, 1.6 g saturated fat | 42.91 g carbohydrate | 16.39 g protein | 160 mg sodium | 4.1 g fiber

The Most Potent Heavy Metal Detoxer

Garlic is one of the single best foods for flushing heavy metals from your body. A potent antioxidant, it fights free radicals that are created when free radicals in your body collide with free radicals in heavy metal pollutants.

Recipes for 30-Day Heavy Metal Detox

Broccoli Salad

Serves: 6

INGREDIENTS

4 cups broccoli, chopped

2 large green onions, sliced

4 celery stalks, chopped

½ cup toasted walnuts, chopped

½ cup raisins

1½ cups plain nonfat yogurt

2 tablespoons seasoned rice vinegar

1 tablespoon honey

Salt and pepper to taste

Combine broccoli, green onions, celery, walnuts, and raisins in large mixing bowl.

Mix yogurt with rice vinegar and honey.

Pour yogurt mixture over broccoli and toss to coat.

Season to taste with salt and pepper.

---

164 calories | 7.7 g fat, 1.4 g saturated fat | 18.3 g carbohydrate | 5.1 g protein | 60 mg sodium | 1.52 g fiber

Crunch on Celery

Celery is loaded with potassium, which helps reduce the inflammation that accompanies toxification. It also helps restore restful sleep.

Recipes for 30-Day Heavy Metal Detox

Turkey Meatballs and Baby Bok Choy

Serves: 4

INGREDIENTS

⅓ cup brown rice, uncooked

1 cup water (to cook rice)

¼ cup green onion, minced

½ pound ground turkey breast

2 egg whites

3 heads baby bok choy

1 cup low-sodium chicken broth

1 cup water

¼ cup low-sodium soy sauce

1 tablespoon light brown sugar

2 teaspoons extra-virgin olive oil

1 garlic clove, minced

1 tablespoon fresh gingerroot, minced

1½ tablespoons dry sherry

2 teaspoons cornstarch

What the Chinese Know about Heavy Metal

Bok choy, or Chinese cabbage, is high in vitamins K and D, both of which are potent antioxidants that fight free radicals from heavy metal pollutants and help boost the immune system.

Cook rice in water. Cool.

Combine rice, green onion, turkey, and egg whites to form meatballs.

Heat oven to 350°F. Place meatballs on sheet tray lined with foil and sprayed with pan spray. Bake for 20 minutes, or until cooked through.

Cut bok choy in half lengthwise and rough chop.

Combine chicken broth, water, soy sauce, and brown sugar.

In large sauce pan, sauté bok choy in olive oil, garlic, and gingerroot, and add stock mixture. Bring to a boil, cover, and reduce heat.

Combine sherry and cornstarch to make a slurry that will thicken the sauce. Stir into saucepan mixture, boil, and then reduce heat.

Serve meatballs in large bowl with sauce poured over them.

476 calories | 11.5 g fat, 2.46 g saturated fat | 47.66 g carbohydrate | 42 g protein | 1000 mg sodium | 4.88 g fiber

Cauliflower Soup

Serves: 4

INGREDIENTS

6 cups cauliflower, chopped

1 teaspoon garlic

Fresh cracked black pepper, to taste

2 cups low-fat, reduced-sodium chicken broth

1 cup medium-sharp Cheddar cheese

1 cup fat-free half-and-half

Steam cauliflower.

Combine cauliflower, garlic, pepper, broth in blender and blend until very smooth. Transfer to saucepan.

Stir in cheese until melted. Finish soup with half-and-half and fresh cracked pepper to taste.

205 calories | 10 g fat, 6 g saturated fat | 15.27 g carbohydrate | 13.38 g protein | 294 mg sodium | 1.34 g fiber

It's All about Sulforaphane

Like Brussels sprouts, cauliflower is high in sulforaphane as well as fiber, both of which help flush heavy metal toxins from the body.

Roasted Cauliflower

Serves: 2

INGREDIENTS

2¼ cups cauliflower, cut into ½-inch florets

½ cup balsamic vinegar

3 tablespoons extra-virgin olive oil

1 teaspoon garlic powder

½ teaspoon kosher salt and fresh cracked black pepper, to taste

Toss cauliflower with balsamic vinegar, oil, and garlic powder.

Place on cookie sheet lined with foil and sprayed with pan spray.

Sprinkle salt and pepper on cauliflower.

Bake at 400°F for 15–20 minutes or until cauliflower is deep brown.

225 calories | 19 g fat, 2.66 g saturated fat | 7.28 g carbohydrate | 2.44 g protein | 576 mg sodium | 1 g fiber

Why You Should Love Cauliflower

Cauliflower stimulates the body's detox systems and helps flush out heavy metal toxins. It also contains the compound allicin, which helps detoxify the blood and liver. Cauliflower is also high in vitamin C, a potent antioxidant.

Recipes for 30-Day Heavy Metal Detox

Mandarin Chicken Salad

Serves: 4

INGREDIENTS

½ cup rice wine vinegar

3 tablespoons dark sesame oil

1 tablespoon low-sodium soy sauce

6 ounces pineapple juice

1 teaspoon gingerroot, minced

1 garlic clove, minced

⅛ teaspoon ground pepper flakes

2 boneless breasts of chicken

Salt and pepper to taste

2 cups napa cabbage, shredded

4 ounces sliced mushrooms

½ cup green onion, sliced

½ cup snow peas, sliced

4 ounces water chestnuts, sliced

1 red bell pepper, seeded and cut into strips

To make dressing whisk together rice wine vinegar, sesame oil, soy sauce, pineapple juice, ginger, garlic, and red pepper flakes.

Rinse chicken and season with salt and pepper. Place on baking pan and roast chicken in 350°F oven until cooked to 160°F internal temperature.

Combine cabbage, mushrooms, green onion, snow peas, water chestnuts, bell pepper, and chicken with salad dressing.

Serve on cold plates.

---

289 calories | 12.5 g fat, 2.1 g saturated fat | 19.46 g carbohydrate | 24.51 g protein | 284 mg sodium | 3.93 g fiber

Peppers Are Absolutely Stimulating!

High in antioxidant vitamins C and A, red peppers help cleanse the arteries and heart muscle, stimulate circulation, and help fight free-radical damage from heavy metal toxins.

Recipes for 30-Day Heavy Metal Detox

Candied Brussels Sprouts

Serves: 2

INGREDIENTS

1½ cups fresh Brussels sprouts, trimmed, cut in half lengthwise

½ cup sugar

1 tablespoon unsalted butter

2 tablespoons apple cider vinegar

Salt and pepper, to taste

Steam Brussels sprouts until tender, about 10 minutes.

Melt sugar in skillet until it turns a light caramel color.

Reduce heat, add butter and vinegar. Caramel will bubble furiously. Stir constantly.

Add Brussels sprouts and reduce heat to low. Cook on low heat until most of the liquid is absorbed and the sprouts are coated with the caramel glaze.

Add salt and pepper to taste.

100 calories | 5.7 g fat, 3.4 g saturated fat | 9.77 g carbohydrate | 2.29 g protein | 73 g sodium | 1 g fiber

Part II: Elimination Detox Diets

Swiss Chard

Serves: 2

INGREDIENTS

⅛ cup pine nuts

¼ cup extra-virgin olive oil

2 large shallots, minced

½ pound Swiss chard, stems removed

Salt and pepper to taste

⅛ cup craisins

A Gift from the Swiss

Swiss chard is one of the most nutrient-rich vegetables. High in fiber, it also has nine times the RDA for vitamin K. Swiss chard is also loaded with many antioxidants that fight free-radical damage.

Toast the pine nuts in oven at 350°F for 5–6 minutes. Watch carefully, as nuts burn quickly.

Sauté shallot in olive oil in large sauté pan.

Add Swiss chard and sauté until limp but still crisp.

Season with salt and pepper.

Place on plate and top with pine nuts and craisins.

369 calories | 32.5 g fat, 4.4 g saturated fat | 13 g carbohydrate | 3.36 g protein | 249 mg sodium | 1.95 g fiber

Part III

Flushing Detox Diets

Whether you've been feasting on French fries or eating your weight in pepperoni pizza, this chapter can help you flush out the excesses. The four diets in this chapter include the 10-Day Cholesterol Flush, the 15-Day Carb Flush, the 7-Day Protein Flush, and the 5-Day Water-Retention Flush. Each diet will help you flush out excess amounts of otherwise essential nutrients that are "clogging up the works" and causing a variety of health problems, from excess water weight and bloating to more serious conditions like high blood pressure and diabetes.

Chapter 9

10-Day Cholesterol Flush

CHOLESTEROL COMES IN TWO VARIETIES: HDL, or "good" cholesterol, and LDL, or "bad" cholesterol. Your liver makes cholesterol, but you also get it from foods you eat, especially from animal protein and saturated fat. While HDL "good" cholesterol is healthy and essential for bodily functions, excess LDL "bad" cholesterol clings to the lining of blood vessels and leads to hardening of the arteries, which may contribute to heart disease and stroke. The 10-Day Cholesterol Flush will help you lose weight and lower your LDL "bad" cholesterol by reducing your total intake of cholesterol and fat.

Close-Up on Cholesterol

A soft waxy substance that circulates along with other fats in your blood, cholesterol is manufactured by the body to build cell membranes, make certain important hormones, including sex and adrenal gland hormones, and ensure the proper functioning of internal organs. You also get cholesterol from certain foods you eat, including fatty meat, butter, cream, and other sources of saturated fat.

High levels of HDL "good" cholesterol scrub the walls of blood cells, flush out excess LDL "bad" cholesterol, and carry it back to the liver so it can be eliminated from the body. Some experts also believe that HDL cholesterol removes excess cholesterol from plaque in arteries, and also inhibits its growth. There are both nondietary and dietary strategies to significantly increase your HDL cholesterol. Nondietary methods include exercising 20–30 minutes a day, stopping smoking, and losing weight. Dietary changes that can help include using more monounsaturated oils, like olive and canola oils in place of polyunsaturated vegetable oils, avoiding partially hydrogenated oils (trans fats), eating more

> ### DETOX TIP
> High cholesterol means your total cholesterol is greater than 200 mg/dL and/or your LDL "bad" cholesterol reading is above 160 mg/dl, which signals an increased risk of heart attack and stroke.

beans, oats, and fruits for their soluble fiber, and eating more foods with omega-3 fatty acids, such as fish and walnuts.

> **Food for Thought**
> *If you have too much LDL cholesterol in your blood, it can cling to artery walls that feed your heart and brain, and form plaque, which could lead to a condition called arteriosclerosis.*

The Best Ways to Cut Total Cholesterol

According to the American Heart Association, there are a few ways you can reduce your total cholesterol. These include:

- Limit your daily fat intake of all fats to between 25 and 35 percent of your daily calories.
- Limit cholesterol intake to 300 milligrams daily.
- Reduce your intake of saturated fats to less than 7 percent of total calories daily.

In addition, you can reduce your cholesterol by making these healthy changes:

- Eliminate all trans fats from your diet, or limit intake to less than 1 percent of total calories daily.
- Avoid commercially fried foods and baked goods made with shortening or partially hydrogenated vegetable oils, including fried fast foods like French fries. Hydrogenated fats, along with trans fats, are the worst culprits when it comes to raising cholesterol.
- Replace saturated fats found in animal products with heart-healthy polyunsaturated and monounsaturated fats found in fish, nuts, seeds, plant oils, and cold-water fish.
- Consume at least 25 to 30 grams of dietary fiber daily, found in whole grains, fruits, vegetables, and legumes, to promote regularity and help "sweep out" saturated fats and cholesterol from your body.

According to the Mayo Clinic, the five foods will help reduce your cholesterol and prevent cholesterol-related heart disease are:

1. **Oats:** Oats and oatmeal contain soluble fiber, which decreases LDL "bad" cholesterol. Consume 10 grams daily, or the amount found in 1½ cups of cooked oatmeal.
2. **Nuts:** Packed with polyunsaturated fats, nuts help maintain healthy, elastic blood vessels. Consume a small handful daily, or about 1½ ounces.
3. **Cold-water fish:** High in omega-3 fatty acids, cold-water fish helps lower blood pressure and reduce heart attacks. Consume salmon, tuna, herring, mackerel, or halibut at least twice a week.
4. **Extra-virgin olive oil:** Olive oil contains high levels of disease-fighting antioxidants that prevent heart disease. Use 2 tablespoons daily.
5. **Foods fortified with stanols:** Stanols are substances found in plants that help prevent cholesterol absorption. Foods fortified with stanols include orange juice, margarine, and yogurt. Consume stanols on a daily basis.

In addition to consuming a healthy diet low in cholesterol and fats, some people may also need to take prescription drugs to lower their cholesterol to a healthy level. Talk to your physician about the many prescription drugs now being used to lower cholesterol.

Meal Plans for 10-Day Cholesterol Flush

By combining this diet plan with regular exercise (shoot for at least 30 minutes of cardio like walking or swimming), you increase your chances of improving your cholesterol profile without having to resort to prescription drugs. But always work with your doctor to arrive at the combination that best suits you.

Day 1

Breakfast
1 cup Oatmeal with Dried Fruit
1 small handful Walnuts
1 cup Low-Fat Milk or Soy Milk
Herbal Tea or Coffee

Lunch
1 serving Apple Bacon Omelet (page 144)
1 cup Baby Spring Mix Salad with Balsamic Vinaigrette
Herbal Tea

Dinner
4 ounces Turkey Meatloaf
½ cup Mashed Sweet Potatoes
1 cup Leafy Green Salad with Oil and Vinegar Dressing
½ cup Steamed Green Beans with Mushrooms
1 cup Mixed Berries with Low-Fat Whipped Cream
Herbal Tea

Day 2

Breakfast
1 cup Steel-Cut Oats with Apples and Cinnamon
1 cup Grapefruit and Orange Slices
1 cup Low-Fat Milk or Soy Milk
Herbal Tea or Coffee

Lunch
1 serving Grilled Chicken and Nectarine Salad (page 145)
1 small Whole Wheat Baguette
½ cup Vegetable Soup
Herbal Tea

Dinner
4 ounces Broiled Salmon
Baked Potato Wedges
1 cup Steamed Broccoli Spears
Mini Cherry Pie
Herbal Tea

Day 3

Breakfast
1 cup Oatmeal with Raisins and Cinnamon
½ cup Yogurt with Nuts and Berries
6 ounces Apple Juice
Herbal Tea

Lunch
1 whole Wheat Sandwich with Grilled Vegetables and Low-Fat Cheese
½ cup Carrot Sticks with Hummus
Herbal Tea

Dinner
1 serving Special Occasion Filet Mignon with Sherry Mushroom Reduction Sauce (page 146)
½ cup Sautéed Spinach
½ cup Steamed Carrots and Sugar Snap Peas
1 Whole Wheat Dinner Roll
½ cup Strawberry-Rhubarb Pudding
Herbal Tea

Meal Plans for 10-Day Cholesterol Flush

Breakfast

¾ cup Granola with Nuts
1 cup Low-Fat Milk or Soy Milk
6 ounces Cranberry Juice

Lunch

1 cup Mixed Vegetable Stir-Fry
¾ cup Brown Rice
1 cup Mixed Green Salad
Herbal Tea

Dinner

1 serving Grilled San Francisco-Style Chicken (page 147)
1 cup Leafy Green Salad with Oil and Vinegar
Grilled Asparagus
½ cup Corn
1 wedge Angel Food Cake with Frozen Mixed Berries Thawed in Their Juices
Herbal Tea

Day 4

Breakfast

1 cup Steel-Cut Oats with Maple and Brown Sugar
1 small handful Almonds
6 ounces Orange Juice
Herbal Tea

Lunch

4 halves Deviled Eggs with Capers (page 148)
1 cup Spinach Salad with Mushrooms and Radishes
1 slice Whole Wheat Toast
Herbal Tea

Dinner

4 ounces Grilled Trout with Citrus Marinade
1 cup Brown Rice Pilaf
1 cup steamed Broccoli, Cauliflower, and Carrots
1 slice Whole Wheat Garlic Bread
½ cup Chunky Homemade Cinnamon Applesauce
Herbal Tea

Day 5

Breakfast

1 cup Multigrain Cereal
1 cup Soy Milk
1 sliced Apple with Peanut Butter
Herbal Tea

Lunch

1 cup Vegetarian Chili Beans with Grated Low-Fat Cheese
2 small Corn Muffins
1 cup Sliced Cucumbers and Radishes with Lime Juice and Chili Powder
Herbal Tea

Dinner

4 ounces Chicken Breast Stuffed with Goat Cheese and Garlic (page 149)
½ cup Roasted Red Potatoes
½ cup Green Peas and Carrots
1 cup Mixed Green Salad
1 Whole Wheat Dinner Roll
½ cup Fruit Salad with a Dollop of Vanilla Yogurt
Herbal Tea

Day 6

Meal Plans for 10-Day Cholesterol Flush

Day 7

Breakfast
1 Southwest Breakfast Burrito with Egg Substitute (2 eggs) Scrambled with Diced Cooked Sweet Potato and Roasted Poblano Chilies
3 tablespoons Tomato or Tomatillo Salsa
1 cup Red Grapes and Watermelon Chunks
1 cup Low-Fat Milk or Soy Milk
Herbal Tea

Lunch
1 Turkey Wrap with Lettuce, Tomato, and Low-Fat Caesar Dressing
1 cup Broccoli, Carrots, Cauliflower, and Red Bell Pepper Marinated in Balsamic Vinaigrette
Herbal Tea

Dinner
4 ounces Baked Italian-Seasoned Pork Tenderloin
1 cup Brown Rice with Artichoke Hearts and Tomatoes
½ cup Corn and Summer Squash Sauté
½ cup Raw Vegetables with Lite Italian Dressing
1 serving Fruit Dip (page 150) with ½ cup Fresh Fruit
Herbal Tea

Day 8

Breakfast
1 cup Oatmeal with Mixed Dried Fruit and Cinnamon
1 cup Low-Fat Milk or Soy Milk
1 small handful Walnuts
6 ounces Pink Grapefruit Juice

Lunch
1 serving Mediterranean Tuna Salad (page 151)
¼ Avocado with Lemon Juice
Herbal Tea

Dinner
4 ounces Beef Fajitas with Peppers and Onions
2 Corn Tortillas
½ cup Mexican Rice
½ cup Seasoned Pinto Beans
½ cup Steamed Zucchini with Cilantro and Low-Fat Cheddar Cheese
Herbal Tea
½ cup Mango Slices with Lime Juice and a Drizzle of Honey

Day 9

Breakfast
1 cup Steel-Cut Oats with Dates and Walnuts
1 cup Low-Fat Milk or Soy Milk
1 cup Blackberries and Sliced Strawberries
Herbal Tea

Lunch
1 medium Whole Wheat Bagel Sandwich with Avocado, Tomato, Onion, and Sprouts
1 cup Fresh Carrot Raisin Salad
Herbal Tea

Dinner
4 ounces Roasted Chicken Breast
½ cup Mashed Potatoes made with Low-Fat Milk and Olive Oil
2 Tomato Halves Broiled with Parmesan and Bread Crumbs
1 cup Mixed Green Salad
1 serving Sweet Ricotta Dessert (page 152)
Herbal Tea

Meal Plans for 10-Day Cholesterol Flush

Breakfast

¾ cup Granola with Fresh
Blueberries

1 cup Low-Fat Milk or Soy
Milk

1 small handful Almonds

6 ounces Orange Juice

Lunch

2 cups Greek Salad with
Romaine, Red Cabbage,
Cucumber, Tomato, Red
Onion, Kalamata Olives,
Feta Cheese, and Lemon-
Garlic Olive Oil Vinaigrette

½ Whole Wheat Pita Bread

¼ cup Hummus

1 Pear

Dinner

1 serving Sesame Citrus
Marinated Scallops (page
153)

1 cup Wild Rice Pilaf

½ cup Steamed Carrots

½ cup Sautéed Spinach

1 Whole Wheat Dinner Roll

½ cup Low-Fat Choco-
late Pudding with Fresh
Raspberries

Herbal Tea

Recipes for 10-Day Cholesterol Flush

Apple Bacon Omelet

Serves: 2

INGREDIENTS

½ cup egg substitute

Salt and pepper to taste

Cooking Spray

¼ cup Canadian bacon, chopped

1 tablespoon low-fat Cheddar cheese

½ Golden Delicious apple, cored and cut into thin strips

Apple of Your Eye

Apples, like all fruits, are a cholesterol-free food that supply lots of nutrients. High in pectin and fiber along with mighty antioxidants such as catechin, quercetin, phloridzin, and chlorogenic acid, new research shows apples help lower LDL "bad" cholesterol and raise HDL "good" cholesterol.

Season egg substitute with salt and pepper.

Spray small sauté pan with cooking spray. Heat pan over medium-low heat and add eggs. Fold gently with heat-safe spatula.

When eggs are nearly cooked add Canadian bacon, Cheddar, and apple and fold over to form omelet shape.

Serve immediately.

---

127 calories | 4 g fat, 1 g saturated fat | 7 g carbohydrate | 14 g protein | 535 mg sodium | 1 g fiber

Recipes for 10-Day Cholesterol Flush

Grilled Chicken and Nectarine Salad

Serves: 2

INGREDIENTS

6 ounces boneless, skinless chicken breasts, grilled

6 ounces romaine lettuce, chopped

⅛ cup low-fat feta cheese, crumbled

½ large nectarine, sliced

¼ cup balsamic vinegar

⅛ cup olive oil

Salt and pepper to taste

The Magic of Citrus

Compounds called limonoids found only in citrus fruits help reduce LDL "bad" cholesterol, raise HDL "good" cholesterol, and help reduce the risk of heart disease.

Grill chicken on hot, well-oiled grill.

Place lettuce in bowl with feta and nectarine slices.

Make dressing by combining balsamic vinegar with olive oil.

Toss greens with dressing and taste. Season with salt and pepper if needed.

Place greens on cold salad plates and top with chicken. Garnish with additional nectarine slices.

---

304 calories | 19.76 g fat, 3.86 g saturated fat | 7.81 g carbohydrate | 23.81 g protein | 136 mg sodium | .73 g fiber

Recipes for 10-Day Cholesterol Flush

Special Occasion Filet Mignon with Sherry Mushroom Reduction Sauce

Serves: 2

INGREDIENTS

2 large shallots, peeled and minced

½ cup mushrooms, sliced

2 tablespoons unsalted butter

½ cup low-sodium beef broth

½ cup dry sherry

1 teaspoon cornstarch

½ cup cold water

12-ounce filet mignon, trimmed of fat

An Elegant Take on Onions

Shallots are low in cholesterol, high in disease-fighting antioxidants, and have the mildest flavor of the onion family, making them ideal for juicing. They also have antibacterial properties that fight infections and skin diseases.

Prepare grill.

Sauté shallots and mushrooms in butter until soft and brown. Add sherry and beef broth and cook until liquid is somewhat reduced.

Thicken sauce by mixing cornstarch with water and stirring into the warm broth mixture. Bring to boil, reduce heat to low.

Season filet with salt and pepper. Grill approximately 4 minutes per side for medium rare. Remove from grill and place on warm plate. Top with mushroom sauce.

467 calories | 24.5 g fat, 12 g saturated fat | 7.83 g carbohydrate | 37.84 g protein | 108 mg sodium | .27 g fiber

Grilled San Francisco–Style Chicken

Serves: 4

INGREDIENTS

1 tablespoon olive oil

1 tablespoon Dijon-style mustard

2 tablespoons raspberry white wine vinegar

Celery salt and pepper to taste

1 small chicken about 2½–3 pounds, cut in quarters

Heat grill to 400°F. In a small bowl, mix the olive oil, mustard, and vinegar. Sprinkle the chicken with celery salt and pepper.

Paint the skin side of the chicken with the mustard mixture. Spray a few drops of olive oil on the bone side.

Grill chicken, bone side to flame, for 15 minutes. Reduce heat to 325°F; cover and cook for 15 minutes.

Mustard More Than Passes Muster

Mustard contains selenium and magnesium—powerful anti-inflammatory agents that help lower high blood pressure, which often accompanies high cholesterol. It also has phytonutrients that inhibit the growth of existing cancer cells and protect against the formation of new ones.

95 calories | 10 g fat | 7 g carbohydrate | 40 g protein | 312 mg sodium | .03 g fiber

Recipes for 10-Day Cholesterol Flush

Deviled Eggs with Capers

Yields: 12 half eggs

INGREDIENTS

6 hard-boiled eggs, shelled and cut in half

½ cup low-fat mayonnaise

1 teaspoon red hot pepper sauce, such as Tabasco

1 teaspoon celery salt

1 teaspoon onion

1 teaspoon garlic powder

1 chili pepper, finely minced, or to taste

2 tablespoons extra small capers

Scoop out egg yolks and place in your food processor along with mayonnaise, seasonings, pepper, and capers. Blend until smooth and spoon into the hollows in the eggs.

Garnish with paprika or chives and chill, covered with aluminum foil tented above the egg yolk mixture.

69 calories | 6 g fat | 0 g carbohydrate | 3 g protein | 235 mg sodium | .11 g fiber

Tiny Capers Pack a Nutritional Wallop

Studies conducted in Italy show that tiny capers, which are actually berries that have been pickled, are packed with natural antioxidants that may help fight heart disease and cancer, especially for those with high cholesterol.

Recipes for 10-Day Cholesterol Flush

Chicken Breast Stuffed with Goat Cheese and Garlic

Serves: 4

INGREDIENTS

4 boneless, skinless organic chicken breasts, rinsed and trimmed of fat

Salt and pepper to taste

1 head garlic

½ cup goat cheese, room temperature

1 teaspoon fresh rosemary, crushed

1 teaspoon fresh thyme

1 tablespoon fresh basil, chopped

¼ cup olive oil

Pan spray

The Good Thing About Garlic

While it probably won't ward off werewolves, garlic is loaded with antioxidants that help lower bad cholesterol, improve cardiovascular health, cleanse the lymph system, and detox the body because of its potent antifungal and antibacterial agents. Numerous studies show that garlic helps decrease LDL "bad" cholesterol and raise HDL "good" cholesterol.

Place chicken between two sheets of plastic wrap and pound thin.

Season with salt and pepper.

Cut top off garlic and drizzle with olive oil. Wrap in foil and bake at 350°F for 1 hour or until garlic is browned (roasted). Cool.

Squeeze roasted garlic out of head and combine with goat cheese and herbs.

Put herb goat cheese mixture on each flattened chicken breast and roll.

Place chicken breasts, seam side down in baking dish sprayed with pan spray. Sprinkle chicken with salt and pepper.

Bake chicken in 350°F oven until internal temperature has reached 165°F. Serve immediately.

---

443 calories | 26.38 g fat, 7.63 g saturated fat | 3.79 g carbohydrate | 47.5 g protein | 229 mg sodium | .31 g fiber

Fruit Dip

Yields: 1½ cups

INGREDIENTS

4 ounces low-fat cream cheese

4 ounces low-fat cottage cheese

1 teaspoon sugar substitute, or to taste

1 teaspoon freshly ground white pepper

2 tablespoons cider vinegar or lemon juice

½ teaspoon salt, or to taste

Blend all ingredients in the blender. Serve chilled.

102 calories | 6.9 g fat | 3.3 g carbohydrate | 6.5 g protein | 508 mg sodium | .07 g fiber

Who Says the Fruit of the Poor Lemon Is Impossible to Eat?

Lemons are high in citric acid and vitamin C. Their high antioxidant content and antibacterial properties help fight conditions related to high cholesterol, including indigestion, constipation, gout, obesity, and blood disorders.

Recipes for 10-Day Cholesterol Flush

Mediterranean Tuna Salad

Serves: 4

INGREDIENTS

12 ounces fresh tuna, rinsed

½ tablespoon Dijon mustard

3 tablespoons sherry vinegar

1 garlic clove, minced

Salt and pepper to taste

2 tablespoons extra-virgin olive oil

4 hard-boiled eggs, peeled, sliced

8 ounces fresh asparagus, steamed

¼ cup red onion, sliced

2 tomatoes, sliced

½ cup kalamata olives, sliced in half

½ cup canned cannellini beans

Broil tuna. Cool and break into chunks.

Whisk mustard, vinegar, garlic, salt, pepper, and olive oil to make salad dressing.

On a large cold plate arrange salad in sections. One section contains the tuna, next to that place eggs, asparagus, onion, tomato, olives, and beans.

Drizzle salad dressing over the top of everything on the plate or pass dressing separately on the side.

388 calories | 24.5 g fat, 4.58 g saturated fat | 11.93 g carbohydrate | 29.89 g protein | 516 mg sodium | 1.63 g fiber

Why Are Beans Good You?

Studies show that beans and other legumes are loaded with dietary fiber, one of the best foods for lowering cholesterol.

Recipes for 10-Day Cholesterol Flush

Sweet Ricotta Dessert

Serves: 1

INGREDIENTS
¼ cup fat-free ricotta cheese
½ teaspoon vanilla extract
1 teaspoon Splenda

Combine ingredients in a bowl, stir well, and enjoy!

---

51 calories | 0 g fat | 4 g carbohydrates | 9 g protein | 120 mg sodium | 0 g fiber

Ricotta Rocks

Ricotta is a delicious, low-calorie, and low-fat source of protein that's also high in calcium, a mineral that helps build strong bones and teeth, and helps you relax, de-stress, and fall asleep.

Recipes for 10-Day Cholesterol Flush

Sesame Citrus Marinated Scallops

Serves: 2

INGREDIENTS

¼ cup fresh lemon juice

¼ cup fresh lime juice

¼ cup fresh orange juice

½ lemon zest

1 tablespoon sugar

1 teaspoon sesame oil

2 teaspoons gingerroot, peeled and finely grated

12 ounces sea scallops, rinsed

2 teaspoons extra-virgin olive oil

Mix citrus juices, zest, sugar, sesame oil, and ginger in small bowl.

Marinate scallops for 10 minutes

Heat olive oil in sauté pan and sear scallops on each side until cooked through.

Set aside. Wipe out skillet and add marinade. Bring to boil and reduce the liquid by half to make sauce. Drizzle sauce on scallops and serve immediately.

Gift from the Sea

High in omega-3 fatty acids, protein, phosphorous, magnesium, and potassium, scallops help lower cholesterol and the incidence of cardiovascular disease and stroke. They also contain cancer-fighting vitamin B12.

347 calories | 8.3 g fat, .9 g saturated fat | 18.1 g carbohydrate | 49.85 g protein | 469 mg sodium | .14 g fiber

Chapter 10

15-Day Carb Flush

STUDIES SHOW LOW-CARB DIETS are the most effective way to shed excess pounds and keep them off. They work by restricting your intake of carbohydrates, especially foods high in sugar and starches, and by keeping you full on low- or no-carb foods like meat, fish, nuts, and produce, so you aren't tempted to cheat on sweets and other carbs. While low-carb diets were once the bane of cardiologists because they encouraged dieters to eat their fill of bacon, burgers, and steak, the latest low-carb diets are heart-healthy alternatives that revolve around unsaturated fats, lean meats, and low-fat or nonfat dairy products.

The Healthy New Way to Low-Carb

Beginning in the late 1970s, studies began showing a high correlation between saturated fats and heart disease, and the low-carb diet appeared doomed. In 2005, Florida cardiologist Arthur Agatston created the South Beach Diet, a heart-healthy version of the Atkins Diet, which breathed new life into low-carb dieting, and gave it the medical stamp of approval.

Dr. Agatston slashed the saturated fat by substituting lean beef, chicken, and fish for fatty meat, and by replacing full-fat dairy products with low- or nonfat versions. Fortunately, low-carb diets also reduce your cravings for sugar and carbs, so you naturally want to eat less of them.

How Low-Carb Diets Work

Low-carb diets help you shed unwanted pounds by reversing an age-old problem called insulin resistance, or the body's inability to properly process fats and sugar. Because humans were genetically designed to store fat to ward off starvation during times of famine, and most people today never encounter famine, people often wind up storing too much fat and become overweight or obese.

Besides helping you lose weight and keep it off, low-carb diets can also put an end to dangerous "yo-yo" dieting. Studies show that going on repeated low-calorie diets lowers your metabolism because your body shifts into starvation mode to preserve fuel. Many obese people are overweight not because they overeat but because repeated dieting has dramatically lowered their metabolism.

Low-carb diets also encourage you to eat until you're satisfied. This relatively novel phenomenon in the world of weight loss has rendered low-carb diets extremely popular.

What You Can and Can't Eat

Healthy foods to consume on a low-carb diet include:

- Fish, especially oily fish such as salmon, tuna, herring, and mackerel, which are loaded with healthy omega-3 fatty acids
- Low-fat or nonfat cheeses and dairy products
- Low-fat or nonfat yogurt
- Leafy greens
- Mushrooms and sprouts
- Chicken and turkey
- Low-fat beef
- Nonstarchy veggies, including celery, radishes, cucumbers, lettuce, cruciferous vegetables, avocadoes, and cucumbers
- Low-carb fruits, including blueberries, raspberries, strawberries, apples, and pears; avoid bananas, citrus fruit, and dried fruit, which are packed with sugar and carbs
- Almonds, walnuts, cashews, seeds, other nuts
- Plant-based vegetable oils, including canola, sunflower, sesame, and olive oil
- Soy products

Stay away from fast foods and commercial snack foods like cake, candy, cookies, French fries, crackers, and chips, all of which are packed with carbs and saturated fats. You should also avoid "white" foods, including foods made with white flour, white rice, potatoes, and white sugar; and low-carb foods with high levels of saturated fat, including hot dogs, bacon, sausage, lunch meat, pork rind, and fatty meats.

Food for Thought

When you are on a low-carb diet, your body begins a process called ketosis which occurs when your intake of carbs is so low that your body is forced to burn fat for fuel instead of carbs. According to Dr. Agatston, ketosis is not dangerous in healthy people, although it may cause dehydration. The most important thing to understand about ketosis is that you don't need to be in it to shed pounds, he says. In fact, a 2006 study published in the American Journal of Clinical Nutrition *concluded that low-carb diets and reduced- or moderate-carb diets were "equally effective in reducing body weight and insulin resistance," but noted that the low-carb diet (ketogenic) resulted in adverse metabolic effects. For this reason, some proponents recommend limiting low-carb diets to 1–2 weeks to "kick start" weight loss and then transitioning to a safer, moderate-carb diet.*

Meal Plans for 15-Day Carb Flush

Many of these meal options call for "sugar-free" options; wherever possible, opt for those that do NOT include artificial sweeteners. Instead look for, or create items that are sweetened with pure maple syrup, brown rice syrup, raw honey, agave syrup, or stevia. For Days 8–15, go to Day 1 and repeat the sequence.

Day 1

Breakfast
Scrambled Egg Burrito (page 160)
½ cup Fresh Blueberries
Herbal Tea or Coffee

Lunch
1 cup Ricotta Spinach Bake (page 196)
1 Low-Fat Whole Wheat Roll
Herbal Tea

Dinner
4-ounce Citrus Grilled Pork Tenderloin (page 161)
1 cup Garlicky Sautéed Green Beans
1 cup Mixed Greens Salad
½ cup Sugar-Free Chocolate Pudding with Sugar-Free Whipped Topping

Day 2

Breakfast
2 (5-inch) Blueberry Pancakes (made with walnut flour) with Sugar-Free Syrup
3 ounces Canadian Bacon
Berries with Heavy Cream
Herbal Tea

Lunch
4 ounces Teriyaki Chicken Satay with Peanut Sauce
1 cup Cabbage Slaw
6 ounces Sugar-Free Lemon-Lime Slush
Herbal Tea

Dinner
1 serving Honey Lime Grilled Chicken (page 162)
1 serving Twice-Baked Sweet Potato (page 163)
1 cup Mixed Green Salad
1 slice Ricotta Cheese Cake with Blueberries and Cream
Herbal Tea

Day 3

Breakfast
1 cup Tofu Scrambled with Spinach (page 22)
½ cup Sugar-Free Yogurt with Strawberries
Herbal Tea

Lunch
1 serving Tuna Cakes with Lemon Sauce (page 164)
1 cup Mixed Spring Greens with Vinegar and Oil
Herbal Tea

Dinner
6 ounces Slow-Cooked Kielbasa with Beer and Sauerkraut
1 cup Collard Greens with Bacon
½ cup Sugar-Free Banana Pudding with Sugar-Free Cookies
Herbal Tea

Meal Plans for 15-Day Carb Flush

Breakfast
3-egg Denver Omelet
1 slice Low-Carb Toast
½ cup Raspberries with a
    Dollop Whipped Cream
Herbal Tea

Lunch
1 cup Stir-Fried Vegetables
⅔ cup Brown Rice
½ cup Cottage Cheese with
    Sugar-Free Preserves
Herbal Tea

Dinner
1 serving Zinfandel-Marinated
    Tri-Tip (page 165)
1 serving Grilled Vegetables
    (page 166)
1 cup Mixed Spring Greens
    with Oil and Vinegar
1 cup Sugar Free Ice Cream
Herbal Tea

Day 4

Breakfast
1 slice Low-Carb Toast with
    Avocado
2 slices Turkey Bacon
Herbal Tea

Lunch
4 ounces Tuna Salad in
    a Low-Carb Wrap with
    Sprouts
1 cup Marinated Mushrooms
Herbal Tea

Dinner
1 cup Fettuccini Alfredo with
    Low-Carb Pasta
½ cup Steamed Broccoli
1 cup Mixed Green Salad
1 serving Darn-Low-Fat Rasp-
    berry Cheesecake (page 167)
Herbal Tea

Day 5

Breakfast
2 Low-Carb Waffles with
    Strawberries and Sugar-
    Free Syrup
½ cup Fat-Free Cottage
    Cheese
Herbal Tea

Lunch
1 (4-ounce) Bunless Cheese-
    burger in a Lettuce Wrap
½ cup Sweet Potato Fries
Herbal Tea

Dinner
1 serving Mahi Mahi over Mixed
    Greens with Lime Wasabi Vin-
    aigrette (page 168)
1 slice Low-Carb Toast with
    Cream Cheese
½ cup Sugar-Free Frozen Yogurt
    with Chopped Walnuts
Herbal Tea

Day 6

Breakfast
3 Scrambled Eggs with Spin-
    ach and Mushrooms
½ cup Sugar-Free Yogurt
    with Blueberries
Herbal Tea

Lunch
1 Ground Beef and Cheese
    Burrito in a Low-Carb
    Tortilla with Lettuce and
    Cilantro
1 cup Cucumber and Rad-
    ish slices with Lime
    Juice, Olive Oil, and Chili
    Seasoning
Herbal Tea

Dinner
1 serving Artichoke-Stuffed
    Chicken Breast (page 169)
1 cup Mashed Cauliflower
½ cup Sautéed Green Beans
    with Garlic
1 (2-inch-square) Low-Carb
    Brownie with Walnuts
Herbal Tea

Day 7

Recipes for 15-Day Carb Flush

Scrambled Egg Burrito

Serves: 2

INGREDIENTS

2 eggs

1 tablespoon water

1 tablespoon unsalted butter

4 tablespoons low-fat Cheddar cheese, shredded

1 teaspoon Italian parsley, chopped

2 low-carb tortillas

1 tablespoon salsa

1 tablespoon light or fat-free sour cream

1 tomato, seeded and chopped

Partial to Parsley

Packed with chlorophyll, vitamins A and C, calcium, magnesium, phosphorous, potassium, sodium, and sulfur, parsley helps stimulate metabolism—a good thing when you're trying to lose weight.

Mix eggs and water together until light and frothy.

Heat butter on medium-low heat and scramble eggs. When eggs are almost cooked add cheese and melt, sprinkle eggs with parsley.

Warm tortilla in microwave for 20 seconds. Add egg to warm tortilla and top with salsa, sour cream, and tomato. Roll up and serve.

252 calories | 10.15 g fat, 3.49 g saturated fat | 24.45 g carbohydrate | 15.72 g protein | 294 mg sodium | .29 g fiber

Citrus Grilled Pork Tenderloin

Serves: 2

INGREDIENTS

½ cup orange marmalade

¼ cup fresh orange juice

Zest of 1 orange

¼ cup fresh lime juice

⅛ cup low-sodium soy sauce

2 large cloves garlic, minced

8 ounces pork tenderloin, trimmed of fat

½ teaspoon coarse-grind black pepper

The Other Skinny Little White Meat

Pork only sounds fattening. In fact, tenderloin has no carbs, and is the leanest cut of pork with a very low fat content. One serving supplies more than half the RDA for thiamin, an essential vitamin for metabolizing carbs, protein, and fat.

Combine marmalade, orange juice, zest, lime juice, garlic, and soy sauce in small saucepan. Heat on medium-low heat until marmalade has liquefied. Remove from heat and cool.

Sprinkle pork tenderloin with black pepper.

Place pork in large ziplock bag with marinade mixture. Marinate overnight.

Grill pork on hot, well-oiled grill until internal temperature has reached at least 150°F. Do not overcook pork, or it will be tough.

Discard marinade.

Allow pork to rest for 5 minutes before slicing.

---

415 calories | 4.3 g fat, 1.4 g saturated fat | 66.45 g carbohydrate | 27.59 g protein | 539 mg sodium | .57 g fiber

Honey Lime Grilled Chicken

Serves: 4

INGREDIENTS

½ cup honey

⅓ cup low-sodium soy sauce

¼ cup fresh lime juice

Zest of 1 lime

¼ cup orange juice

Zest of 1 orange

Black pepper

4 boneless, skinless chicken breasts

The Joy of Soy Sauce

New research shows uncooked soy helps lower LDL "bad" cholesterol by up to 9 percent by increasing the enzyme activity that helps break down cholesterol. If you're trying to lower your cholesterol as well as lose weight, stock up on soy sauce!

Combine honey, soy sauce, lime juice and zest, orange juice and zest, and black pepper.

Place chicken in marinade and put in large plastic bag.

Marinate for at least 1 hour and up to 24 hours.

Grill chicken on hot, well-oiled grill until it is cooked through.

Discard marinade.

---

374 calories | 4.85 g fat | 38.94 g carbohydrate | 43.64 g protein | 739 mg sodium | .08 g fiber

Twice-Baked Sweet Potatoes

Serves: 4

INGREDIENTS

2 large sweet potatoes, scrubbed

2 ounces fat-free cream cheese

2 tablespoons skim milk

1 teaspoon cinnamon

1 tablespoon brown sugar

¼ cup pecan pieces

The Fiber Has It

Potatoes are packed with fiber, which help reduce cholesterol, and promote regularity. This low-fat recipe uses fat-free cream cheese instead of butter to reduce saturated fats, which help lower cholesterol.

Heat oven to 400°F.

Wash and pierce potatoes. Bake 30–40 minutes, or until soft.

Cut potatoes in half lengthwise and scoop the potato out.

Mix cream cheese with potatoes, milk, cinnamon, and brown sugar until well blended.

Spoon cream cheese potato mixture back into potato shells and sprinkle pecans on top.

Bake 8–10 minutes or until potatoes are heated through and nuts are brown.

205 calories | 8.3 g fat, 2.5 g saturated fat | 28.75 g carbohydrate | 3.88 g protein | 74 mg sodium | 3.88 g protein | 2 g fiber

Recipes for 15-Day Carb Flush

Tuna Cakes with Lemon Sauce

Serves: 4

INGREDIENTS
½ cup whole wheat bread
12 ounces cooked tuna fillet
¼ cup green onion, minced
2 large egg whites
1 teaspoon lemon pepper
1 teaspoon garlic powder
½ cup Smart Beat mayonnaise
1 tablespoon fresh dill weed
Zest of 1 lemon
Juice of 1 lemon
Black pepper to taste

Toast bread and cool. Tear into cubes.

Combine tuna, bread crumbs, green onions, egg white, lemon pepper, and garlic powder.

Form into 4 patties.

Bake 350°F for 25 minutes or until golden brown and set.

Make sauce using mayonnaise, dill, lemon zest, and lemon juice. Season with black pepper.

Serve tuna cake with lemon sauce.

Cholesterol Benefits of Tuna and Dill

Studies show tuna and salmon are packed with omega-3 fatty acids, which help lower LDL "bad" cholesterol) and raise HDL "good" cholesterol. Dill weed is rich in antioxidants and dietary fibers that also help control blood cholesterol levels.

170 calories | 4.55 g fat, 1.1 g saturated fat | 9.75 g carbohydrate | 22.56 g protein | 313 mg sodium | .34 g fiber

Recipes for 15-Day Carb Flush

Zinfandel-Marinated Tri-Tip

Serves: 6

INGREDIENTS

1 cup red Zinfandel wine

½ cup brown sugar

¾ cup onion, thinly sliced

1 tablespoon minced garlic

1 tablespoon gingerroot, peeled and thinly sliced

½ teaspoon coarse-grind black pepper

½ teaspoon mustard

2 pounds beef tri-tip roast

Mix wine, brown sugar, onion, garlic, gingerroot, pepper, and mustard together.

Place tri-tip in large ziplock bag with marinade.

Marinate overnight.

Grill tri-tip on hot, well-oiled grill. Let meat rest for 5 minutes before slicing. Slice against grain into thin slices.

Discard marinade.

269 calories | 8.42 g fat, 2.93 g saturated fat | 13.15 g carbohydrate | 36.26 g protein | 90 mg sodium | .21 g fiber

Try Tri-Tip

Lower in fat than other cuts of beef, and containing zero carbs, tri-tip is the perfect meat to marinade. High in omega-3 fatty acids, beef is one of the best sources of CLA (conjugated linoleic acid), another healthy fat. Studies on laboratory animals showed that CLA reduced the incidence of cancer, and suppressed the growth of existing cancers.

Recipes for 15-Day Carb Flush

Grilled Vegetables

Serves: 4

INGREDIENTS

1 tablespoon minced garlic

2 tablespoons extra-virgin olive oil,

2 tablespoons balsamic vinegar

2 medium red onions, cut into round slices

2 medium red bell peppers, cut into 2-inch wide strips

2 medium yellow squash, cut into ½-inch slices

2 large zucchini, cut into ½-inch slices

Kosher salt and black pepper to taste

Combine garlic, olive oil, and balsamic vinegar.

Place vegetables in a large bowl and coat with vinegar mixture.

Sprinkle with salt and pepper.

Prepare grill and cook vegetables on high heat.

Sprinkle with additional salt and pepper if desired.

156 calories | 7.99 g fat, 1.1 g saturated fat | 17.42 g carbohydrate | 3.5 g protein | 567 mg sodium | 1.5 g fiber

Shed Pounds Without Feeling Hungry!

The vegetables in this dish will fill you up without filling you out. All super-low in carbs, squash and zucchini are high in B vitamins and niacin, calcium, and potassium, while onions and red peppers are packed with disease-fighting antioxidants.

Darn Low-Fat Raspberry Cheesecake

Serves: 8

INGREDIENTS

3 (8-ounce) packages fat-free cream cheese, softened

¾ cup Splenda

1 teaspoon vanilla extract

¾ cup Egg Beaters

1½ cups frozen raspberries

1 prepared low-fat graham cracker crust

In an electric mixer, combine cream cheese, Splenda, and vanilla on medium speed. Add Egg Beaters and mix until well blended.

Gently fold raspberries into mixture. Pour mixture into crust. Bake at 350°F for 40 minutes or until center is almost set.

Cool and refrigerate for 2 hours or overnight.

238 calories | 8 g fat | 31 g carbohydrates | 15 g protein | 645 mg sodium | 1 g fiber

Berry RX

Eating a diet rich in raspberries as well as blueberries, cranberries, and strawberries may help to reduce your risk of several types of cancer. Raspberries also contain lutein, which is important for healthy vision. Berries contain less carbs than other fruits, so enjoy a handful when you get a craving.

Recipes for 15-Day Carb Flush

Mahi Mahi over Mixed Greens with Lime Wasabi Vinaigrette

Serves: 2

INGREDIENTS

12 ounces Mahi Mahi, rinsed

2 tablespoons extra-virgin olive oil, divided

1 teaspoon lemon pepper

1 tablespoon wasabi

1 tablespoon low-sodium soy sauce

1 tablespoon rice wine vinegar

1 teaspoon sesame oil

6 ounces mixed greens

Eat More, Lose More

Low in carbs and high in vitamins, leafy greens help you shed unwanted pounds by filling you up on very few calories. Eating lots of leafy greens can also lower your cholesterol and reduce your risk of heart attack. The best veggies for fighting cholesterol include dark green veggies like spinach, kale, collard greens, and Swiss chard.

Brush Mahi Mahi with 1 tablespoon olive oil. Sprinkle lemon pepper on fish. rill Mahi Mahi on well-oiled grill until fish is cooked through; approximately 4 minutes per side.

To make wasabi dressing, combine wasabi, soy sauce, and vinegar. Whisk in sesame oil and olive oil. Reserve some of the dressing to drizzle on the fish.

Mix greens with wasabi dressing until well coated.

Place greens on large plate and top with grilled fish.

Drizzle additional dressing on fish.

---

277 calories | 14.82 g fat, 2.39 g saturated fat |6.38 g carbohydrate | 29.57 g protein | 752 mg sodium | .35 g fiber

Artichoke-Stuffed Chicken Breast

Serves: 2

INGREDIENTS

2 (5-ounce) boneless, skinless chicken breasts,

Salt and pepper to taste

2 ounces artichokes hearts

¼ cup reduced-fat Monterey jack cheese, thinly sliced

1 tablespoon extra-virgin olive oil

¼ cup seasoned breadcrumbs,

½ small white onion, finely diced

½ cup mushrooms, sliced

½ cup dry white wine

An Oldie but Goodie

One of the oldest known cultivated vegetables on earth, artichokes contain cynarin, a substance that has been shown to lower LDL "bad" cholesterol. Its high fiber content helps detox the intestines, and promote regularity. Artichokes are also rich in disease-fighting antioxidants, including vitamin C and folic acid, and contain healthy carbs that help regulate blood sugar levels.

Rinse chicken and pat dry.

Flatten chicken using mallet by placing chicken between two sheets of plastic wrap. Season with salt and pepper.

Place artichoke hearts on top of each chicken breast and top with slice of cheese.

Roll chicken and place seam side down in baking dish that has been sprayed with pan spray.

Sprinkle salt and pepper on outside of chicken breasts. Drizzle with olive oil. Sprinkle breadcrumbs on top. Place onions, mushrooms, and wine in baking dish surrounding the chicken.

Bake at 350°F covered with foil for 35–45 minutes, or until chicken is done.

366 calories | 13.8 g fat, 3.7 g saturated fat | 17 g carbohydrate | 43.4 g protein | 331 mg sodium | .81 g fiber

Chapter 11

7-Day Protein Flush

PROTEIN IS FOUND IN A WIDE VARIETY OF FOODS. The highest amount is found in meat, fish, eggs, poultry, milk, cheese, and yogurt, which all contain about 8 grams of protein per serving. Cereals and grains provide about 2 grams of protein per ½ cup or slice, and vegetables have about 1 gram per half cup. Although protein is necessary to grow, maintain, and repair bodily tissues, and to help the body battle infections and heal wounds, consuming too much protein can overload the kidneys and force it to work too hard. Studies show protein overload can also lead to obesity, dehydration, acidosis, and other health problems. The 7-Day Protein Flush will help you safely reduce your intake of protein. If you suffer from kidney or liver disease, consult with your physician before following any low-protein diet.

Health Benefits of a Low-Protein Diet

Reducing your intake of protein can help you lose weight by reducing your intake of saturated fat. If you have a family history of gout, which is caused by an excess of uric acid in the blood, a low-protein diet can also help reduce your risk of it. In addition, studies show that a low-protein diet may also reduce symptoms in Parkinson's disease.

Reducing protein can also help your kidneys. Although your kidneys comprise only about 0.5 percent of your total body weight, more than 20 percent of your blood goes through them for cleansing and other functions. Even if you don't have kidney disease, consuming too much protein can tax your kidneys and inhibit normal kidney functioning, which includes:

- Maintaining a healthy composition of your blood
- Maintaining a healthy electrolyte balance in the body
- Regulating the volume of water in your body
- Removing toxic wastes from your body, including urea, ammonia, drugs, and other toxic substances

- Maintaining a constant acid/alkaline balance in your blood
- Helping control your blood pressure
- Stimulating the manufacturing of blood cells
- Regulating healthy calcium levels

How to Eat a Low-Protein Diet

You should never completely eliminate protein from your diet, even when you're following a low-protein diet. Protein helps increase thermogenesis, or the amount of calories your body burns, and also helps your body burn fats. Consuming too little protein forces the body to steal essential amino acids (the building blocks of protein) from muscles and other tissues. Because the body is basically metabolizing itself, this process, called catabolism, can lead to muscle loss and weakness.

The easiest way to reduce your protein intake is to eliminate or dramatically reduce your intake of meat, fish, poultry, eggs, and dairy products. Fortunately, this book offers you four delicious options, including The 5-Day Protein Flush, the 15-Day Vegan Detox, the 10-Day Raw Food Detox, and the 15-Day Mediterranean Detox.

You can lower your daily consumption of protein by using commercial low-protein products available through Dietary Specialties (888-640-2800 or *www.info@dietspec .com*). The company manufactures low-protein breads, crackers, cookies, pasta, baking mixes, cheese sauces, and other foods.

> **Food for Thought**
> *If you're suffering from weight gain, fluid retention, bloating, constipation, a bad taste in the mouth, nausea, headaches, and fatigue, you may be consuming too much protein.*

Meal Plans for 7-Day Protein Flush

Once you've completed your 7-Day plan, you'll want to begin incorporating protein back into your diet. Ideally, you'll only want to eat a palm-size portion of protein (about 3 to 6 ounces) at any one meal. Balance that with healthy, non-refined carbohydrates, you'll get the perfect metabolic mix!

Breakfast

Stuffed Peach French Toast
  (page 175)
Mixed Berries with Whipped
  Cream
Herbal Tea or coffee

Lunch

Bean Salad with Vinaigrette
  (page 176)
1 Fresh Peach or Nectarine
Herbal Tea

Dinner

1 cup Veggie Stroganoff with
  Portobello Mushrooms
1 cup Noodles
½ cup Steamed Broccoli
1 Dinner Roll
Herbal Tea

Day 1

Breakfast

1 slice Whole Wheat Toast
  and Avocado
1 cup Blueberries
6 ounces Orange Juice
Herbal Tea or Coffee

Lunch

Barley Salad with Almonds
  (page 177)
½ cup Sautéed Zucchini and
  Red Bell Pepper Strips
6 ounces Cranberry Juice

Dinner

2 ounces Shrimp Stir-Fried
  with Snow Peas
1 cup White Rice
Garden Salad with Olive Oil
  and Lemon Dressing
1 serving Dark Chocolate–
  Covered Berries (page 178)
Herbal Tea

Day 2

Breakfast

2 Banana Pancakes with
  Sliced Strawberries
6 ounces Cranberry Juice
Herbal Tea

Lunch

1 serving Granola (page 179)
  with Sliced Banana
1 cup Low-Fat Milk or Soy
  Milk
Herbal Tea

Dinner

1½ cups Spaghetti Squash
  with Marinara Sauce
1 cup Mixed Green Salad
  with Oil and Vinegar
1 slice Garlic Bread
½ cup Fresh Pineapple
  Chunks with Shredded
  Coconut
Herbal Tea

Day 3

Meal Plans for 7-Day Protein Flush

Day 4

Breakfast
1 cup Crispy Rice Cereal with Sliced Banana
½ cup Low-Fat Milk or Soy Milk
6 ounces Orange Juice

Lunch
2 cups Greek Salad with Lemon, Garlic, and Olive Oil
1 sliced Pear with a Dollop of Vanilla Yogurt
Herbal Tea

Dinner
1 cup Stir-Fried Spinach Seasoned with Garlic and Soy Sauce
1 cup White Rice
1 serving Balsamic-Glazed Carrots (page 180)
Herbal Tea

Day 5

Breakfast
2 pieces Banana Bread with Cream Cheese
1 sliced Orange
Herbal Tea

Lunch
1 cup Vegetable Curry with Potatoes and Carrots
½ Pita Bread
½ cup Sliced Cucumbers and Tomatoes with Lemon Juice
½ cup Mixed Berries
Herbal Tea

Dinner
1 cup Baked Eggplant Parmesan with Marinara Sauce
1 cup Steamed Broccoli with Lemon
1 cup Mixed Green Salad with Italian Vinaigrette
1 slice Garlic Bread
3 Ultimate Low-Fat, Low-Protein Chocolate Chip Cookies (page 180)
Herbal Tea

Day 6

Breakfast
1 cup Cream of Wheat Cereal
1 slice Toast with Avocado
6 ounces Cranberry Juice
Herbal Tea

Lunch
1 ounce Turkey on Whole Wheat Bread with Lettuce and Tomato
½ cup Baked Sweet Potato Fries
Herbal Tea

Dinner
1 serving Mediterranean-Style Penne (page 181)
1 cup Mixed Spring Greens Salad with Vinegar and Oil
1 slice Garlic Bread
1 Baked Apple with Cinnamon
Herbal Tea

Day 7

Breakfast
1 medium Cinnamon Raisin Bagel with Cream Cheese
1 cup Cantaloupe Chunks with Blackberries
Herbal Tea

Lunch
1 serving Green Bean, Cucumber, and Potato Salad (page 182)
1 small French Baguette with Butter
½ cup Sliced Peaches
Herbal Tea

Dinner
2 Marinated Grilled Vegetable Kebobs
1 cup White Rice with Parsley
½ cup Sautéed Spinach with Garlic
1 Dinner Roll
½ cup Coffee Frozen Yogurt
Herbal Tea

Recipes for 7-Day Protein Flush

Stuffed Peach French Toast

Serves: 6

INGREDIENTS

1 French bread loaf, cut into 1-inch thick slices

4 ounces light cream cheese, softened

4 tablespoons peach preserves

2 large peaches, peeled and sliced

4 eggs

1 cup half-and-half

1 teaspoon pure vanilla extract

Peaches Promote Health (If Not Immortality)

Peaches have no protein, but are high in phytonutrients and antioxidants, which help reduce heart disease, cancer, arthritis, and eye ailments. For those on a low-protein diet (under 40 milligrams daily), peaches are a sweet treat you can enjoy to your heart's content.

Preheat oven to 350°F.

Cut a pocket in the bottom crust of each piece of bread. Take care not to slice it all the way through.

Mix cream cheese and preserves together. Fold in peaches.

Stuff peach cream cheese mixture into each slice of bread.

Beat eggs, half-and-half, sugar, and vanilla together.

Spray the bottom of a 13″ × 9″ glass baking dish.

Place bread slices in baking dish and pour egg mixture over. Make sure that all bread is covered with the egg mixture.

Bake uncovered for 30–45 minutes.

Remove from oven, cool slightly, and sprinkle with powdered sugar.

433 calories | 14.73 g fat, 7 g saturated fat | 58.46 g carbohydrate | 16.52 g protein | 599 mg sodium | .49 g fiber

Recipes for 7-Day Protein Flush

Bean Salad with Vinaigrette

Serves: 4

INGREDIENTS

½ pound green beans, trimmed

8 ounces low-sodium garbanzo beans, rinsed

1 cup cherry tomatoes, sliced in half

¼ cup green onion, tops included, thinly sliced

½ cup marinated artichoke hearts, drained

2 tablespoons Italian flat-leaf parsley, minced

¼ cup pitted kalamata olives, cut in half

1 teaspoon Dijon mustard

⅓ cup red wine vinegar

¼ cup balsamic vinegar

1 tablespoon minced garlic

¼ cup walnut oil

Salt and pepper to taste

Combine beans, tomatoes, green onion, artichokes, parsley, and olives in large bowl.

Make dressing by combining Dijon, vinegars, and garlic. Whisk in walnut oil until thick. Pour over bean mixture.

Toss bean mixture well and taste. Season with salt and pepper if needed.

259 calories | 21 g fat, 2.65 g saturated fat | 11.72 g carbohydrate | 5.8 g protein | 683 mg sodium | 2.65 g fiber

The Skinny on Garbanzos

With a nutty flavor and crunchy texture, garbanzo beans are a great addition to any salad. Packed with fiber, they help lower cholesterol. Unlike animal protein, which comes bundled with saturated fat and cholesterol, the protein in garbanzo beans is fat free and heart healthy.

Recipes for 7-Day Protein Flush

Barley Salad with Almonds

Serves: 4

INGREDIENTS

2 tablespoons extra-virgin olive oil

1 tablespoon unsalted butter

1 cup barley

1 tablespoon minced garlic

1 cup water

2 cups low-fat, low-sodium chicken broth

½ cup dry roasted almonds

Salt and pepper to taste

Heat olive oil and butter in large sauté pan. Mix in barley and stir until barley is toasted brown (about 5 minutes).

Add garlic, water, and chicken broth and bring to a boil. Lower heat to a simmer.

Cook until barley is tender and liquid has been absorbed.

Remove from heat and add almonds. Taste and add salt and pepper if necessary. Serve immediately.

I'm Just Wild about Barley

Barley is a nutritious grain that lends a nutty flavor and chewy texture to foods. High in fiber and containing no fat or cholesterol, it helps lower LDL "bad" cholesterol, and reduce the risk of heart disease.

399 calories | 20 g fat, 3 g saturated fat | 45.26 g carbohydrate | 9.2 g protein | 42 mg sodium | 1.3 g fiber

Dark Chocolate–Covered Berries

Serves: 2

INGREDIENTS
½ cup dark chocolate
1 teaspoon shortening
8 large strawberries

Melt chocolate over a double boiler.

Add shortening and stir well.

Dip strawberries in chocolate and place on parchment paper.

Refrigerate until chocolate is set.

282 calories | 17.43 g fat, 8.7 g saturated fat | 31 g carbohydrate | 2.48 g protein | 15 mg sodium | 3.5 g fiber

Another Excuse to Eat Chocolate

Dark chocolate is packed with disease-fighting phytochemicals, as well as flavonoids that promote healthy heart function. Studies show that eating dark chocolate may prevent hardening of the arteries, which could lead to a heart attack.

Recipes for 7-Day Protein Flush

Granola

Serves: 12

INGREDIENTS

¾ cup unsalted butter, melted

¾ cup maple syrup

2 teaspoons vanilla extract

2 teaspoons cinnamon

4 cups old-fashioned rolled oats

1 cup chopped pecans

1 cup wheat germ

1 cup raisins

Feeling Your Oats

Considered a superfood, oats lower total choles-terol, reduce the risk of heart disease and stroke, and are packed with soluble fiber that cleanses your intestines. Oats are also rich in vitamin E, an antioxidant that fights free radicals, which trigger cancers; selenium, which boosts immunity and improves mood; and B vitamins, which provide energy.

Preheat oven to 325°F.

Combine butter, maple syrup, vanilla, and cinnamon.

Place oats, pecans, and wheat germ in a large bowl and stir in butter mixture until well coated.

Bake granola for 20 minutes, stirring halfway through.

Bake until mixture is crisp and golden brown.

Cool and stir in raisins.

---

404 calories | 20 g fat, 8 g saturated fat | 47.81 g carbohydrate | 7.52 g protein | 7 mg sodium | 4.1 g fiber

Recipes for 7-Day Protein Flush

Balsamic-Glazed Carrots

Serves: 2

INGREDIENTS

2 cups carrots

2 tablespoons extra-virgin olive oil

1 tablespoon unsalted butter

1 tablespoon brown sugar

Salt and pepper to taste

1½ tablespoons balsamic vinegar

Sauté carrots in olive oil and butter until tender. Add brown sugar and stir until sugar is dissolved.

Season with salt and pepper.

Add balsamic vinegar and cook until carrots are tender.

Serve immediately.

234 calories | 18.7 g fat, 5.2 g saturated fat | 15.17 g carbohydrate | 1.1 g protein | 59 mg sodium | 1.7 g fiber

Ultimate Low-Fat, Low-Protein Chocolate Chip Cookies

Serves: 12

INGREDIENTS

Betty Crocker Chocolate Chip Cookie Mix

¼ cup Egg Beaters

½ cup Smart Squeeze or ½ cup sugar-free vanilla-flavored syrup

Preheat oven to 350°F. Coat two large cookie sheets with nonstick spray and set aside.

Mix all ingredients in a large bowl with a fork until moist and smooth. Using a teaspoon, drop cookie dough onto sheets without crowding.

Bake for 8 to 10 minutes.

122 calories | 3 g fat | 21 g carbohydrates | 1 g protein | 87 mg sodium | 0 g fiber

Sneaky Fun

These cookies are completely deceptive. No one in the world would ever believe they are low in fat. In fact, it might be fun for you to serve them to your friends and family and wait until the raves come in to tell them that they're really a healthier version of original chocolate chip cookies.

Mediterranean-Style Penne

Serves: 4

INGREDIENTS

2 tablespoons canola oil

1 medium eggplant, diced

12 medium mushrooms, quartered

2 tablespoons minced garlic

2 tablespoons minced shallots

4 ounces dry white wine

2 tablespoons capers

4 cups pitted kalamata olives, chopped

1 tablespoon balsamic vinegar

1 tablespoon tomato paste

1 pound penne pasta, cooked

4 ounces feta cheese, crumbled

¼ cup Italian flat-leaf parsley, minced

Heat oil in large skillet. Add eggplant and reduce heat to medium. Cook for 5 minutes, stirring occasionally. Add mushrooms, garlic, and shallots. Cook for an additional 5 minutes, stirring. Add white wine, capers, olives, vinegar, and tomato paste. Simmer for 5 minutes.

Add pasta to hot water to rehydrate and warm. Drain and add to skillet with vegetables.

Serve on warm plate and garnish with feta and parsley.

523 calories | 15 g fat, 5.3 g saturated fat | 76.69 g carbohydrate | 20 g protein | 693 g sodium | 2.4 g fiber

The World's Most Edible Fungus

Mushrooms, like many vegetables, have no protein, but plenty of other nutrients, including folic acid, niacin, copper, and significant amounts of potassium. Studies show the potassium in mushrooms helps maintain fluid balance in the body, aids muscle and nerve function, and regulates heart rhythm.

Recipes for 7-Day Protein Flush

Green Bean, Cucumber, and Potato Salad

Serves: 4

INGREDIENTS
½ pound green beans, trimmed
5 red potatoes, quartered
2 large cucumbers, peeled and sliced
3 celery stalks, sliced
¼ cup red wine vinegar
¾ cup light mayonnaise
Salt and pepper to taste

What's in a Cuke Besides Water?

They might seem too tasteless to be nutritious, but cucumbers are actually a good source of dietary silica, a mineral of emerging importance that may protect against Alzheimer's disease. They are also high in iodine, which regulates the thyroid gland and helps the body utilize fats to protect against obesity. Like most vegetables, cucumbers have no protein.

Blanch green beans by placing in boiling water for 3 minutes and then putting into a bowl of ice water.

Cook potatoes in large pot of water until tender.

Mix potatoes, green beans, cucumbers, and celery in large bowl.

Combine red wine vinegar and mayonnaise to make salad dressing. Pour over potato mixture. Taste and season with salt and pepper.

---

431 calories | 9 g fat, 1.6 g saturated fat | 78 g carbohydrate | 8.5 g protein | 417 mg sodium | 3.9 g fiber

Chapter 12

5-Day Water Retention Flush

RETAINING WATER IS NO FUN. Suddenly you can't zip up your favorite jeans, or you feel like a caricature of yourself because your face is so puffy. Water retention can be caused by many factors, including heart and kidney problems, circulation problems, and lack of exercise because of an extended injury or illness. Some medications can also cause bloating and water retention. The 5-Day Water Retention Flush addresses the most common cause of water retention, which is consuming too much sodium.

Drowning in Sodium

According to the National Academy of Sciences' Institute of Medicine, the average person requires from 1,500 to 2,400 milligrams of salt daily, depending on weight and activity level, or how much you sweat out. According to the American Dietetic Association, most Americans consume five times more salt than required for bodily functions, or more than 10,000 milligrams of salt daily!

Which isn't to suggest that sodium is a bad thing. Everyone needs a small amount of sodium for health and bodily function. Consumed in moderation, sodium plays many roles in the body, including:

- Helping the body maintain a proper balance of fluids
- Assisting with the transmission of nerve impulses throughout the body
- Regulating muscle contraction and relaxation

> **Food for Thought**
> *Even if you think you only use a pinch or dash of salt to flavor your foods, you're probably consuming far more sodium than you realize. Studies show just 11 percent of the sodium in the typical American diet comes from the salt shaker. The rest, or 77 percent, is disguised in processed and prepared foods, some of which may not taste the least bit salty (so you add even more salt)!*

What Causes Water Retention?

When you consume too much sodium, it begins collecting in your blood. Because sodium hangs on to water, your blood volume goes up, which forces your heart to pump harder to move more blood through your blood vessels. The result is bloating, fluid retention, water-weight gain, and accompanying irritation, headaches, depression, and high blood pressure. Low-calorie and especially low-fat diets below 1,200 calories a day can also cause water retention because they don't contain enough protein to draw excess water from your tissues.

Sometimes, water retention can be caused by consuming too little fluids. Because you become dehydrated, your body overcompensates by holding on to fluids. Other causes of water retention include:

- High levels of female hormones, especially estrogen and progesterone, which results in swelling in the tummy and breasts. (This explains why many women suffer from PMS and water retention around their menstrual periods.)
- Antihistamines, which make cells leak water and protein into tissues.
- Some medications, including antibiotics.
- Poor digestion, which can lead to changes in your intestine that release histamines.

Sleuthing Out the Salt

In general, most Americans get their salt from three sources:

Processed and prepared foods: Canned vegetables, soups, lunch meats, and frozen foods are loaded with salt or sodium compounds, which are used as preservatives and to enhance the food's taste and texture. A bowl of canned chicken broth contains nearly 800 milligrams of sodium or more than half the RDA for sodium for some people.

Condiments that contain sodium: Table salt isn't the only culprit when it comes to sodium content. Although 1 teaspoon provides a whopping 2,325 milligrams of sodium, other condiments are even higher, including soy sauce, which contains 1,000 milligrams of sodium! Other high-sodium condiments include ketchup, mustard, salsa, relish, pickles, olives, and salad dressings.

Some foods come by their sodium content naturally. Meat, dairy products, poultry, and vegetables all contain moderate amounts of sodium. Just 1 cup of low-fat milk provides 110 milligrams of sodium.

Tuna fish, tomato sauce, bagels, packaged and processed foods, and prepared foods like pepperoni pizza, hot dogs, bacon, ham, seasoned rice, French fries, and macaroni and cheese, are also high in sodium.

Sodium is also found in monosodium glutamate (MSG), baking powder, baking soda, disodium phosphate, sodium nitrate, sodium alginate, and nitrate. If you're on a low-sodium diet, don't forget to read the food labels!

How to Shake the Salt Habit

The easiest way to decrease your sodium intake is to become a food detective and read food labels to determine sodium content. And don't forget to do the math! Some food labels provide sodium content per package, and that package may have two or three servings.

Plenty of foods contain less than 150 milligrams of salt. They include wine, coffee, tea, soft drinks, bread, cake, cookies, cereals, crackers, pasta, butter, margarine, oil, ice cream, sherbet, half-and-half, milk, all fresh fruits and vegetables, frozen fruits and vegetables prepared without sauces, and low-sodium canned vegetables or rinsed canned veggies. Certain cheeses, including mozzarella, ricotta, and Monterey jack are also low in sodium.

> **DETOX TIP**
>
> Some of your favorite foods may already be low in salt, so don't think you have to sacrifice taste to cut the sodium.

All unprocessed meats, poultry, and fish are also low in sodium, as are eggs, peanut butter, and unsalted snacks like unsalted nuts and popcorn. Don't think you have to sacrifice taste to cut the sodium; some of your favorite foods may already be low in salt:

- Grill up a steak on the barbeque for only 50 milligrams. Just watch the BBQ sauce, which is high in salt.
- Enjoy your steak with a baked potato, which has just 5 milligrams of sodium.
- Have a sliced tomato salad. One tomato supplies just 50 milligrams of sodium.

In addition to the 5-Day Water Retention Flush, the 15-Day Carb Flush also acts as a natural diuretic and will help you eliminate excess water.

Meal Plans for 5-Day Water Retention Flush

It goes without saying that you should stay away from salting your food as you work through this plan, but it can be a hard habit to break! In lieu of blindly adding table salt to your dishes, try using herbs to flavor your food instead. If you really crave the salt, go for pure sea salt (splurge on Himalayan) as it contains beneficial natural minerals.

Day 1

Breakfast
1 cup Oatmeal with Raisins and Cinnamon
1 cup Low-Fat Milk or Soy Milk
6 ounces Orange Juice
Herbal Tea or Coffee

Lunch
1 serving Mushroom Spinach Frittata (page 188)
1 serving Summer Tomato Salad (page 189)
Herbal Tea

Dinner
4 ounces Broiled Salmon Marinated in Citrus Juices and Olive Oil
½ cup Mashed Sweet Potatoes
1 cup Spinach Salad with Mushrooms, Oil, and Vinegar
1 Whole Wheat Dinner Roll
½ cup Frozen Yogurt with Sliced Strawberries
Herbal Tea

Day 2

Breakfast
2 Scrambled Eggs
1 slice Whole Wheat Toast with Fruit Preserves
½ cup Cranberry Juice
Herbal Tea or Coffee

Lunch
1 cup Pasta with Garlic, Broccoli, Pine Nuts, Olive Oil, and Lemon Juice
1 cup Leafy Green Salad with Mushrooms, Tomatoes, and Radishes
Herbal Tea

Dinner
1 serving Grilled Chicken with Fresh Tomato Salsa (page 190)
½ cup Coleslaw
½ cup White Rice
1 serving Blueberry Peach Cobbler (page 191)
Herbal Tea

Day 3

Breakfast
1 cup Steel-Cut Oatmeal with Slivered Almonds
1 cup Low-Fat Milk or Soy Milk
½ cup Sliced Peaches
Herbal Tea

Lunch
1 serving Spinach Orange Salad (page 192)
2 ounces Turkey Breast and Avocado Wrap
Herbal Tea

Dinner
1 serving Shrimp Kebabs with Lemon Slices (page 193)
½ cup Brown Rice with Cashews and Green Onion
½ cup Grilled Asparagus
1 cup Mixed Spring Greens Salad with Balsamic Vinaigrette
Herbal Tea

Meal Plans for 5-Day Water Retention Flush

Breakfast

1 medium Cinnamon Raisin Bagel with Low-Fat Cream Cheese

1 cup Low-Fat Milk or Soy Milk

½ cup Sliced Bananas and Oranges

Herbal Tea

Lunch

1 serving Butternut Squash Soup (page 194)

1 serving Autumn Coleslaw with Apples and Craisins (page 195)

Herbal Tea

Dinner

1 cup White Bean, Kale, Potato Soup

1 small Whole Wheat Baguette

1 cup Baby Spring Greens Salad with Radishes and Tomatoes

1 cup Sliced Strawberries with Low-Fat Whipped Topping

Herbal Tea

Day 4

Breakfast

2 Poached Eggs on 1 Slice Whole Wheat Toast

½ cup Cantaloupe with Blueberries and a Dollop of Yogurt

1 cup Low-Fat Milk or Soy Milk

Herbal Tea

Lunch

1 serving Ricotta Spinach Bake (page 196)

1 cup Cucumber, Tomato Salad with Apple Cider Vinaigrette

Herbal Tea

Dinner

1 serving Balsamic-Glazed Chicken (page 197)

1 cup Sautéed Swiss Chard with Mushrooms and Red Bell Pepper

1 cup Mashed Potatoes

1 Whole Wheat Dinner Roll

½ cup Raspberry Sorbet with Crushed Pineapple

Herbal Tea

Day 5

Mushroom Spinach Frittata

Serves: 4

INGREDIENTS

1 small onion, diced

1 teaspoon extra-virgin olive oil

10 ounces fresh spinach

½ teaspoon nutmeg

4 eggs

1 cup skim milk

1 teaspoon flour

¼ teaspoon black pepper

½ cup Swiss cheese, shredded

Flush with Onions

Onions contain natural diuretic properties that help flush out excess water, so eat up!

Sauté onion in olive oil.

Add spinach and nutmeg and sauté until liquid has evaporated.

Beat eggs with milk. Add flour and pepper.

Spray a glass pie pan with pan spray and add onion-spinach mixture. Sprinkle cheese on top.

Pour egg mixture over.

Bake 325°F, uncovered for 25–35 minutes, or until frittata is firm and slightly puffed in the center.

218 calories | 12.3 g fat, 4.95 g saturated fat | 9.49 g carbohydrate | 17.23 g protein | 213 mg sodium | .8 g fiber

Recipes for 5-Day Water Retention Flush

Summary Tomato Salad

Serves: 4

INGREDIENTS

4 large heirloom tomatoes

Pepper to taste

2 teaspoons fresh basil, minced

2 tablespoons fresh parsley, minced

½ red onion, thinly sliced

2 stalks celery

1 teaspoon Dijon mustard

4 teaspoons balsamic vinegar

2 cloves garlic, minced

½ teaspoon sugar

2 tablespoons extra-virgin olive oil

1 teaspoon toasted walnuts, chopped

1 teaspoon blue cheese, crumbled

Slice tomatoes into thin slices and place on individual plates. Add pepper, basil, and parsley to top of tomatoes. Add red onion and celery.

Combine Dijon, balsamic vinegar, garlic, sugar, and olive oil to form dressing.

Drizzle dressing over tomato mixture and top with walnuts and blue cheese.

---

145 calories | 8.8 g fat, 1.28 g saturated fat | 13.83 g carbohydrate | 2.57 g protein | 214 mg sodium | 1.8 g fiber

A Very Smart Nut

With only 3 grams of salt per serving, walnuts are low in sodium and high in omega-3 fatty acids, including alpha-linoleic acid (ALA), which improves artery function after a high-fat meal. Studies show walnuts may be even better at lowering cholesterol than olive oil!

Recipes for 5-Day Water Retention Flush

Grilled Chicken with Fresh Tomato Salsa

Serves: 2

INGREDIENTS

1 tablespoon fresh oregano, minced

½ cup fresh lemon juice and 1 teaspoon zest

1 tablespoon extra-virgin olive oil

1 tablespoon Dijon mustard

1 tablespoon Italian flat-leaf parsley, minced

½ teaspoon fresh thyme, minced

½ teaspoon garlic powder

1 cup tomato, washed, seeded, diced small

¼ cup fresh basil, minced

1 tablespoon fresh orange juice and 1 teaspoon zest

1 teaspoon minced garlic

½ red onion, diced small

1 teaspoon balsamic or red wine vinegar

2 (5-ounce) boneless, skinless chicken breasts

Combine oregano, lemon juice, zest, olive oil, Dijon, parsley, thyme, and garlic powder to make marinade. Pour marinade over chicken.

Cover and chill for at least 1 hour and up to 24 hours.

Preheat grill for chicken.

Combine tomato, basil, orange juice, zest, garlic, onion, and balsamic vinegar to make salsa.

Discard marinade and grill chicken until cooked through and juices run clear.

Place chicken on plate and top with salsa.

379 calories | 18.93 g fat, 4.2 g saturated fat | 10.16 g carbohydrate | 42 g protein | 286 mg sodium | 1.5 g fiber

More Than Just a Hot Tomato

Another natural diuretic, tomatoes help rid your body of excess water. They are also high in disease-fighting antioxidants.

Blueberry Peach Cobbler

Serves: 10

INGREDIENTS

6 ripe peaches, blanched in boiling water, skinned and sliced

½ cup fresh lemon juice

1 cup sugar, divided

1 pint blueberries, rinsed and picked over, stems removed

½ cup unsalted butter, melted

½ teaspoon salt

1½ cups rice flour or quinoa flour

1 tablespoon baking powder

1 cup buttermilk

Preheat the oven to 375°F. Slice peaches into bowl and sprinkle with lemon juice and ½ cup sugar. Add the blueberries and mix well.

Prepare a 9" × 13" baking dish with nonstick spray. Spread the peaches and blueberries on the bottom. Pour the melted butter into a large bowl. Add the remaining ½ cup sugar and salt and whisk in the flour and baking powder. Add the buttermilk and stir; don't worry about lumps.

Drop the batter by tablespoonfuls over the fruit. Bake for 35–40 minutes. Cool for 25 minutes. Serve with vanilla ice cream or whipped cream.

"Gold of the Incas"

Quinoa isn't a grain, but a seed that's related to spinach. When cooked, it has a creamy texture that's a cross between polenta and risotto and a nutty flavor. Naturally low in sodium, quinoa is a complete protein and is also rich in lysine, an amino acid that builds and repairs tissue. Quinoa was first discovered by the Incas, who fed it to their warriors to keep them strong in battle.

306 calories | 9.9 g fat | 51.27 g carbohydrate | 2.92 g protein | 306 mg sodium | .78 g fiber

Recipes for 5-Day Water Retention Flush

Spinach Orange Salad

Serves: 2

INGREDIENTS

¼ cup fresh orange juice

¼ cup raspberry vinegar

1 tablespoon honey

1 tablespoon fresh lime juice

¼ teaspoon chili powder

¼ cup extra-virgin olive oil

6 ounces baby spinach

¼ cup red onion, chopped

½ avocado, cubed

⅛ cup jicama, peeled and cut into strips

1 orange, sliced

Whisk orange juice, vinegar, honey, lime juice, chili powder, and olive oil together to make salad dressing.

Place spinach on cold plate and top with red onion, avocado, jicama, and orange slices. Drizzle dressing over top.

493 calories | 39 g fat, 5.4 g saturated fat | 30.36 g carbohydrate | 4.64 g protein | 76 mg sodium | 2.38 g fiber

What the Heck Is Jicama?

Jicama (hick-a-ma) looks like a potato, tastes like an apple, and has the same texture as a radish. Although some call it a Mexican potato, it's actually a legume. High in fiber and potassium and ultralow in sodium, studies show jicama helps lower high blood pressure and cholesterol levels.

Recipes for 5-Day Water Retention Flush

Shrimp Kebabs with Lemon Slices

Serves: 2

INGREDIENTS

1 large lemon, zest and juice

1 lime, zest and juice

2 teaspoons garlic

Fresh cracked pepper to taste

2 teaspoons extra-virgin olive oil

8 large shrimp peeled and deveined

1 large lemon cut into small wedges

Combine lemon juice, lemon zest, lime juice, and lime zest with garlic, pepper, and olive oil. Marinate shrimp for 10 minutes in this mixture.

Thread the shrimp on the skewers, alternating with slices of lemon.

Grill on hot, well-oiled grill brushing with marinade mixture. Shrimp cooks quickly, so watch it carefully.

The Mighty Shrimp

High in potassium as well as zinc, manganese, and calcium, studies show shrimp help lower high blood pressure, which may be caused by consuming too much sodium. Shrimp also protect against Alzheimer's disease, cancer, and heart arrhythmia, and help reduce depression and stabilize mood.

230 calories | 6.28 g fat, 1.09 g saturated fat | 7.51 g carbohydrate | 35.96 g protein | 378 mg sodium | .36 g fiber

Recipes for 5-Day Water Retention Flush

Butternut Squash Soup

Serves: 8

INGREDIENTS

1 large butternut squash, peeled, seeded and cut into chunks

8 cups low-sodium chicken broth

½ teaspoon extra-virgin olive oil

½ onion, diced

1 Granny Smith apple, diced

¼ cup honey

1 pinch nutmeg

½ teaspoon cinnamon

Salt and pepper to taste

Bring squash and broth to boil.

Heat olive oil in skillet and sauté onion and apple until soft.

Add to squash and simmer until squash is tender. Add honey, nutmeg, cinnamon, salt, and pepper.

Cool and then puree in blender until smooth.

172 calories | 1.46 g fat, .13 g saturated fat | 35.29 g carbohydrate | 4.37 g protein | 147 mg sodium |3 g fiber

The High Math of Low-Sodium Products

One easy way to cut salt from your diet is to substitute low-sodium broths for regular products that are notoriously high in sodium. A half cup of regular chicken broth packs in 768 milligrams of sodium, while low-sodium broth contains 538 milligrams.

Recipes for 5-Day Water Retention Flush

Autumn Coleslaw with Apples and Craisins

Serves: 6

INGREDIENTS

¾ cup Smart Beat mayonnaise

⅓ cup light sour cream

2 teaspoons cider vinegar

1 tablespoon maple syrup

1 pound cabbage, shredded

2 Granny Smith apples, cut into thin strips

2 Red Delicious apples, cut into thin strips

1 cup dried cranberries

2 celery stalks, chopped

Salt and pepper to taste

Combine mayonnaise, sour cream, cider vinegar, and syrup to make dressing.

Place cabbage, apples, craisins, and celery in large bowl and toss with dressing.

Season with salt and pepper to taste.

---

214 calories | 2.7 g fat, .55 g saturated fat | 44.65 g carbohydrate | 2.7 g protein | 137 mg sodium | 5.02 g fiber

Ricotta Spinach Bake

Serves: 6

INGREDIENTS

1 medium onion, finely chopped

3 tablespoons unsalted butter

10 ounces frozen chopped spinach, thawed and squeezed dry

½ teaspoon nutmeg

Salt and pepper, to taste

4 eggs, beaten

1 cup low-fat ricotta cheese

½ cup low-fat, low-sodium mozzarella cheese, grated

½ cup Parmigiano-Reggiano cheese, grated

Preheat oven to 350°F.

Sauté onion in butter. Mix in spinach, nutmeg, salt, and pepper. Sauté until all moisture is absorbed. Cool.

Beat eggs with ricotta cheese.

Fold in spinach mixture.

Pan spray a glass pie dish. Pour mixture in and sprinkle mozzarella and Parmigiano-Reggiano cheeses over the top.

Bake 25–30 minutes, or until mixture is set in the center and a toothpick comes out clean.

Strong to the Low-Sodium Finish

Fresh spinach is low in sodium and high in potassium, a combo that's the first line of defense against water retention and high blood pressure. It is also rich in folic acid, which reduces the risk of high blood pressure. Steer clear of canned spinach. Like most canned vegetables, it is very high in sodium.

262 calories | 17.5 g fat, 9 g saturated fat | 7.9 g carbohydrate | 18 g protein | 360 mg sodium | .62 g fiber

Balsamic-Glazed Chicken

Serves: 2

INGREDIENTS

2 (5-ounce) boneless, skinless chicken breasts

Salt and pepper, to taste

2 large cloves garlic

1 teaspoon brown sugar

¼ cup balsamic vinegar

1 tablespoon extra-virgin olive oil

Extra-Virgin

Extra-virgin olive oil is made in a cold-pressed, chemical-free process, which results in a very low-acid oil with a fresh, light taste. Olive oil is ideal for a low-sodium diet, as it contains heart-healthy omega-3 fatty acids that help lower blood pressure and LDL "bad" cholesterol.

Rinse chicken breasts, pat dry, and season with salt and pepper.

Make marinade by combining garlic, brown sugar, balsamic vinegar, and olive oil.

Place chicken in marinade and marinate overnight.

Prepare grill. Remove chicken from marinade and grill until cooked through and the juices run clear. Discard marinade.

---

266 calories | 10.56 g fat, 2 g saturated fat | 4.64 g carbohydrate | 35.56 g protein | 86 mg sodium | .13 g fiber

Part IV

Organ Detox Diets

Your liver, gallbladder, and intestinal tract are continually filtering out dietary and environmental toxins. But your detox organs were never designed to handle the twenty-first century's onslaught of toxins. As a result, your detox organs are forced to work overtime to cleanse your body, which subjects them to constant stress. The three detox diets in this chapter, including the 7-Day Liver Detox, the 10-Day Gallbladder Detox, and the 5-Day Intestinal Detox, provide your detox organs with essential nutrients that help them rest, recharge, and recuperate. In fact, you may want to use these detox diets whenever you feel sluggish or run down.

Chapter 13

7-Day Liver Detox Diet

YOUR LIVER IS RESPONSIBLE FOR THOUSANDS OF ENZYME SYSTEMS that control nearly every activity in your body. If it fails to make just one of those essential enzymes, metabolic imbalances result can result that lead to serious conditions and diseases. Unfortunately, the twenty-first-century lifestyle isn't easy on your liver. Many pollutants and toxins, including environmental toxins, food additives, pesticides, cosmetics, household cleansers, pharmaceuticals, over-the-counter drugs, artist materials, garden chemicals, building supplies, and everyday stress, can destroy liver cells and lead to a variety of health conditions.

Your Liver and Your Life

The largest, and in many ways, the most complex organ in your body, your liver is responsible for breaking down toxic substances absorbed from the intestines or manufactured anywhere else in the body, and eliminating them as harmless substances into the bile.

Your liver also controls thousands of enzyme systems that regulate nearly every activity in your body.

- It acts as a holding tank for vitamins, minerals, and sugars the body uses for fuel.
- Your liver removes toxins from your blood.
- It regulates the production and elimination of cholesterol.

> **DETOX TIP**
>
> Your liver manufactures about 80 percent of your body's cholesterol, much of which is used to make bile. Although too much cholesterol is unhealthy, your body needs an adequate amount to manufacture estrogen, testosterone, and the adrenal hormones. (See the 10-Day Cholesterol Flush, page 137 for more information.)

When your liver becomes imbalanced, it becomes less efficient at eliminating toxins from the body.

How to Detox Your Liver

You can help detox your liver by consuming a diet that eliminates foods that cause an allergic reaction, such as gluten and lactose. Your liver can also become imbalanced if you consume a diet that's too high in acidic foods. Avoiding excess caffeine and alcohol and quitting smoking can also promote healthier liver function.

When you're not consuming enough nutrients, you burden your liver and this can cause a buildup of toxins. To nourish your liver and promote healthy detoxification, consume plenty of the following nutrients:

Folic acid, found in spinach, asparagus, broccoli, kale, cabbage, and blackberries.

Iron, found in blackberries, chard, beets, carrots, pineapple, cauliflower, broccoli, parsley, strawberries, and parsley.

Magnesium, found in beets, broccoli, blackberries, garlic, beet greens, spinach, carrots, cauliflower, parsley, celery, and garlic.

Selenium, found in garlic, oranges, chard, radishes, grapes, carrots, and cabbage.

Vitamin B12, found in lean meats, poultry, fish, and fortified soymilk.

B6 (niacin), found in wheat bran, peanuts, chicken, turkey, and fish.

B2 (riboflavin), found in collard greens, kale, parsley, broccoli, and prunes.

Pantothenic acid, found in cauliflower, kale, and broccoli.

Inositol, found in oranges, grapefruit, peaches, cantaloupe, watermelon, strawberries, tomatoes, and cabbage.

You can also protect your liver by consuming foods that are high in disease-fighting antioxidants, which fight free radicals that damage tissue. Antioxidants are also contained in liver enzymes that help detox the body.

Eight Power Foods for Your Liver

In addition, the following eight power foods will help promote healthy liver function.

1. **Apples:** The pectin in apples binds to heavy metals, and helps the liver eliminate them.
2. **Garlic:** Helps the liver eliminate mercury, food additives, and estrogen from the body, and also contains allicin, a sulfur compound that helps the liver detoxify.
3. **Bitter leafy greens:** The bitter substances in rocket lettuce, chicory, and endive trigger the flow of bile in the liver, and aid digestion and detoxing.
4. **Cruciferous vegetables:** Contain substances that neutralize several toxins found in cigarette smoke (nitrosamines) and peanuts (aflatoxin). Cruciferous veggies also contain glucosinolates, which facilitate the liver's production of detox enzymes.
5. **Artichokes:** Increase the production of bile by 100 percent, and contain substances that act as blood purifiers, which help the liver reduce cholesterol, triglycerides, and other toxic wastes.
6. **Beets:** Contain a substance that purifies the blood and absorbs heavy metals. (See the 30-Day Heavy Metal Detox (page 115) for more information on nutrients that help displace heavy metals.)
7. **Fruits high in antioxidants:** Oranges, grapefruit, apples, pears, berries, prunes, and raisins are packed with antioxidants that fight free radicals, and help promote the health of your liver.
8. **Lemon juice in hot water:** Drink a glass before breakfast every morning to purify the liver, promote regularity, and assist the liver's cleansing actions.

Meal Plans for 7-Day Liver Detox

Beyond this detox, you will continue to tonify and strengthen your liver if you make it a habit to work the liver "Power Foods" into your weekly plan. In addition, your liver will thank you if you cut out most alcohol, caffeine, and processed, fried, or fatty foods from your diet.

Day 1

Breakfast
1 serving Artichoke Cheese Omelet (page 206)
1 slice Whole Wheat Toast with Sugar-Free Preserves
6 ounces Orange Juice
Herbal Tea or Coffee

Lunch
1 serving Tabbouleh Salad with Almonds (page 207)
1 cup Cantaloupe and Watermelon Chunks
Herbal Tea

Dinner
4 ounces Roasted Chicken
½ cup Wild Rice Pilaf
½ cup Sautéed Swiss Chard with Onion, Garlic, and Olive Oil
1 cup Baby Spring Greens Salad
Baked Apple
Herbal Tea

Day 2

Breakfast
1 medium Whole-Grain Bagel with Almond Butter
½ cup Papaya Chunks with 1 cup Vanilla Yogurt
Herbal Tea

Lunch
1 serving Romaine and Watercress Salad with Sunflower Seeds (page 208)
1 cup Miso Soup with Tofu
Herbal Tea

Dinner
4 ounces Vegetarian Meatloaf
½ cup Carrot Salad with Lemon-Olive Oil Dressing
½ cup Roasted Belgian Endive
Frozen Yogurt with Berries and Whipped Cream
Herbal Tea

Day 3

Breakfast
2 small Sweet Potato Pancakes with Lite Sour Cream
1 Hardboiled Egg
½ cup Chunky Homemade Applesauce with Cinnamon
Herbal Tea

Lunch
1 Hummus Wrap with Cucumber, Tomatoes, and Yogurt Dressing
1 cup Sliced Carrots Marinated in Lemon Juice and Olive Oil
2 small Plums
Herbal Tea

Dinner
1 serving Stuffed Cabbage Rolls (page 209)
½ cup Boiled Red Potatoes with Olive Oil, Garlic, and Parsley
1 cup Mixed Green Salad
½ cup Mango Sorbet
Herbal Tea

Meal Plans for 7-Day Liver Detox

Breakfast

1 cup Steel-Cut Oatmeal
 with Dried Fruit
1 cup Low-Fat Milk or Soy
 Milk
1 Sliced Orange
Herbal Tea

Lunch

1 cup Stir-Fried Vegetables
 with 2 ounces Shrimp
½ cup Brown Rice
1 ounce Dark Chocolate
Herbal Tea

Dinner

1 serving Grilled Chicken
 Taco Salad (page 210)
1 cup Grilled Pineapple and
 Apricot Halves with a Dol-
 lop of Crème Frâiche
Herbal Tea

Day 4

Breakfast

2 Eggs Scrambled with
 Tomatoes and Mushrooms
1 serving Baked Grapefruit
 (page 210)
1 slice Whole Wheat Toast
Herbal Tea

Lunch

1 cup Vegetarian Vegetable
 Soup
1 medium French Roll, Split
 and Filled with Lite Tuna
 Salad
Herbal Tea

Dinner

4 ounces Roast Beef
1 serving Artichoke Rice Pilaf
 (page 211)
½ cup Roasted Cauliflower
1 cup Garden Salad with
 Apple Cider Vinaigrette
½ cup Blueberry Crisp
Herbal Tea

Day 5

Breakfast

2 medium Whole Wheat
 Banana Pancakes with
 Sliced Strawberries
2 ounces Canadian Bacon
6 ounces Orange Juice
Herbal Tea

Lunch

2 cups Baby Spring Greens
 Salad with Fresh Roasted
 Beets, Goat Cheese, and
 Balsamic Vinaigrette
1 small Whole Wheat
 Baguette
Herbal Tea

Dinner

4 ounces Roast Pork Tenderloin
½ cup Low-Fat Scalloped
 Potatoes
1 serving Lemon-Glazed
 Brussels Sprouts (page 212)
1 cup Garden Salad
2-inch-square Low-Fat
 Brownie with Walnuts
Herbal Tea

Day 6

Breakfast

1 cup Yogurt with Fresh
 Peaches, Bananas, and
 Walnuts
1 slice Rye Toast with
 Avocado
6 ounces Tomato Juice
Herbal Tea

Lunch

1 cup Lo Mein Noodles with
 Stir-Fried Snow Peas and
 Carrots
½ cup Broccoli Marinated
 with Flax Seed Oil and Soy
 Sauce
Herbal Tea

Dinner

1 serving Chicken Satay
 Skewers (page 213)
1 cup Brown Rice
1 serving Mixed Pepper
 Salad with Balsamic Dressing (page 214)
½ cup Stir-Fried Baby Bok Choy
½ Banana Split Lengthwise
 and Broiled with Honey
 and Walnuts
Herbal Tea

Day 7

Artichoke Cheese Omelet

Serves: 2

INGREDIENTS

2 eggs

Salt and pepper to taste

1 tablespoon unsalted butter

⅓ cup canned artichoke hearts, drained and chopped

2 tablespoons low-fat Cheddar cheese, grated

2 tablespoons reduced-fat Monterey jack cheese, grated

1 tablespoon Parmesan cheese, grated

1 tablespoon light sour cream

Whisk eggs until thick and frothy. Season with salt and pepper.

Heat butter on medium low in a nonstick pan. Scramble softly using a heat safe spatula. Stir in artichokes, Cheddar, and Monterey jack.

Cook until eggs are done. Sprinkle with Parmesan cheese.

Serve with a dollop of sour cream.

283 calories | 19.88 g fat, 8.79 g saturated fat | 5.72 g carbohydrate | 20.2 g protein | 362 mg sodium | .35 g fiber

Why Are Artichokes So Important for Your Liver?

Artichokes are a liver superfood because they increase the production of bile by 100 percent, which in turns promotes healthy digestion.

Recipes for 7-Day Liver Detox

Tabbouleh Salad with Almonds

Serves: 4

INGREDIENTS

1 cup boiling water

1 cup cracked bulgur wheat

¼ cup fresh lemon juice

⅓ cup extra-virgin olive oil

4 cloves garlic, minced

¼ teaspoon kosher salt and freshly ground black pepper

1 cucumber, peeled, seeded, and diced

2 tablespoons parsley, minced

1 tablespoon fresh mint, minced

4 green onions, including tops, sliced

1 red bell pepper, seeded and diced

½ cup almonds, roasted

Pour 1 cup boiling water over cracked wheat; cover with plastic, and let sit for 20 minutes or until liquid is absorbed.

For the dressing whisk lemon juice, olive oil, garlic, salt, and pepper.

Add cucumber, parsley, mint, green onion, and red bell pepper to cracked wheat mixture. Toss with dressing. Stir in almonds.

This salad may be served immediately or refrigerated for 2 days.

448 calories | 27.99 g fat, 3.44 g saturated fat | 39.55 g carbohydrate | 9.41 g protein | 156 mg sodium | 2.1 g fiber

Focus on Bulgur

Bulgur wheat is a protein-packed grain that has no fat or cholesterol, which can lead to a "fatty liver." The garlic in this recipe also helps cleanse your liver.

Recipes for 7-Day Liver Detox

Romaine and Watercress Salad with Sunflower Seeds

Serves: 2

INGREDIENTS

1½ cups romaine lettuce, chopped

1 cup watercress, chopped

1 teaspoon Dijon mustard

2 tablespoons raspberry vinegar

Salt and pepper to taste

2 tablespoons extra-virgin olive oil

⅛ cup sunflower seeds, dry roasted

A Salad That Promotes a Healthy Liver

Romaine lettuce and watercress are high in beta-carotene and vitamin A, which help support the liver. Sunflower seeds and extra-virgin olive oil provide a healthy dose of essential fatty acids, which also promote a healthy liver.

In a large bowl combine lettuce and watercress.

Whisk together mustard, vinegar, and salt and pepper. Drizzle in olive oil whisking until the dressing becomes thick.

Pour dressing over the greens and season to taste.

Serve salad on cold plates and garnish with a sprinkle of sunflower seeds.

150 calories | 14.76 g fat, 1.95 g saturated fat | 2.78 g carbohydrate | 1.46 g protein | 345 mg sodium | .4 g fiber

Recipes for 7-Day Liver Detox

Stuffed Cabbage Rolls

Serves: 4

INGREDIENTS

1 large head green cabbage

½ cup white rice, cooked

½ pound extra-lean ground beef

Salt and pepper to taste

½ teaspoon dried thyme

½ onion, diced small

1 cup low-sodium tomato juice

½ cup low-sodium beef broth

1 (16-ounce) can diced tomatoes

½ cup sauerkraut, rinsed, drained

1 tablespoon cornstarch

1 cup cold water

What Are Glucosinolates?

Substances called "glucosinolates" in cruciferous veggies like cabbage (and sauerkraut) facilitate the liver's production of enzymes, which helps it cleanse and detoxify the body.

Steam cabbage until leaves are pliable. Plunge into bowl of ice water to stop the cooking. Cut off the core end and gently pull leaves off in one piece. Try not to tear them.

In large bowl combine rice, ground beef, salt, pepper, thyme, and onion.

Make a small test patty and cook to make sure the seasoning is correct.

Fill each cabbage leaf with the ground beef mixture. Secure closed with toothpick.

Place cabbage leaves in large Dutch oven and cover with tomato juice, beef broth, and diced tomatoes. Cover and steam until beef is cooked through.

Add sauerkraut and cook sauce for 10 additional minutes.

Remove cabbage rolls from pot. Mix cornstarch and water together in a small cup and add to the sauce. Bring to a boil and stir, reduce heat. Sauce will thicken.

Top with the tomato sauce and serve.

348 calories | 11 g fat, 4 g saturated fat | 42.51 g carbohydrate | 19.65 g protein | 484 mg sodium | 2.75 g fiber

Grilled Chicken Taco Salad

Serves: 2

INGREDIENTS

5 cups romaine lettuce, shredded

6 ounces organic, boneless, skinless chicken breast

½ cup no-salt kidney beans, rinsed, drained

½ cup light sour cream

½ large avocado, mashed

2 large tomatoes, diced

½ cup salsa

¼ cup low-fat Cheddar cheese, shredded

Rinse chicken. Pat dry and season. Grill on hot, well-oiled grill until cooked.

Cool chicken and cube or shred for salad.

Mix salsa, avocado, and sour cream together for salad dressing.

Toss lettuce with dressing until leaves are evenly coated. Place on cold plates and top with chicken and tomatoes.

484 calories | 22 g fat, 5.95 g. saturated fat | 32.49 g carbohydrate | 37.83 g protein | 433 mg sodium | 4.21 g fiber

Baked Grapefruit

Serves: 4

INGREDIENTS

2 tablespoons dark brown sugar

2 pink grapefruit, cut in half, sections cut through

2 tablespoons brandy

2 teaspoons pecan halves, toasted and chopped

Pat brown sugar into each grapefruit halves.

Pour brandy on top and cover with plastic. Refrigerate overnight.

Broil for 5 minutes or until bubbly and light golden brown.

Top with pecan pieces before serving.

79 calories | 2.36 g fat, .2 g saturated fat | 13.52 g carbohydrate | .93 g protein | 1 mg sodium | .5 g fiber

Recipes for 7-Day Liver Detox

Artichoke Rice Pilaf

Serves: 2

INGREDIENTS

½ cup marinated artichoke hearts
1 cup brown rice, uncooked
1 teaspoon extra-virgin olive oil
1 cup water
1 cup low-sodium chicken broth
¼ cup Italian parsley, minced

Another Reason to Love Artichokes

Artichokes contain substances that act as blood purifiers and that help the liver break down cholesterol, triglycerides, and other toxic wastes.

Drain artichokes and set aside.

In a large skillet sauté rice in olive oil over low heat unless rice becomes golden. Place water and chicken broth in saucepan and bring to boil. Add rice. Cover, reduce heat to low. Cook until rice is done, approximately 40–45 minutes.

Fluff with fork, stir in artichokes and parsley.

Serve immediately.

216 calories | 1.8 g fat, .37 g saturated fat | 44.16 g carbohydrate | 5.9 g protein | 215 mg sodium | 5 g fiber

Lemon-Glazed Brussels Sprouts

Serves: 2

INGREDIENTS

2 cups fresh Brussels sprouts, trimmed and cut in half

1 lemon, juice and zest

3 tablespoons light brown sugar

1 tablespoon Dijon mustard

1 tablespoon unsalted butter

Salt and pepper to taste

¼ cup cashews, lightly salted, chopped

Steam Brussels sprouts until tender, approximately 15 minutes.

Add lemon juice, zest, sugar, mustard, and butter to large frying pan. Cook until bubbling. Add Brussels sprouts and stir well. Season with salt and pepper to taste.

Serve with cashews sprinkled on top.

317 calories | 19.61 g fat, 8.56 g saturated fat | 28.76 g carbohydrate | 6.41 g protein | 211 mg sodium | 1.6 g fiber

Why Do Brussels Sprouts Detoxify Your Liver?

Cruciferous veggies like Brussels sprouts have substances that neutralize several toxins found in cigarette smoke (nitrosamines) and peanuts (aflotoxin), both of which infiltrate your liver and may cause liver disease.

Recipes for 7-Day Liver Detox

Chicken Satay Skewers

Serves: 2

INGREDIENTS

¼ cup onion, diced

½ cup low-fat plain yogurt

1 tablespoon extra-virgin olive oil

1 teaspoon fresh gingerroot, peeled and grated

½ teaspoon ground cumin

1 teaspoon ground turmeric

¼ teaspoon salt and pepper

1 large clove garlic, minced

12 ounces organic, boneless, skinless chicken breast, rinsed and cut into ½-inch-wide and 4-inch-long strips suitable for placing on a skewer.

Combine all ingredients except chicken in blender to make marinade.

Place chicken in large ziplock bag with marinade. Seal and marinate for at least 2 hours and up to 24 hours.

Soak wooden skewers for 30 minutes.

Thread pieces of chicken onto each skewer; placing 1 strip per skewer.

Heat and oil grill. Grill chicken until cooked through.

Discard marinade.

---

327 calories | 12.5 g fat, 2.8 g saturated fat | 7.83 g carbohydrate | 45.83 g protein | 422 mg sodium | .34 g fiber

How Does Yogurt Help Your Liver?

The active-culture yogurt helps repopulate your liver and digestive tract with organisms that help break down food, while the acidophilus in yogurt encourages healthy bacterial growth in the liver, and helps reduce the production of bile acid, which may contribute to cancer.

Recipes for 7-Day Liver Detox

Mixed Pepper Salad with Balsamic Dressing

Serves: 4

INGREDIENTS

1 cup red onion, diced small

2 cloves garlic, minced

2 carrots, peeled and diced small

3 tablespoons extra-virgin olive oil

2 yellow bell peppers, seeded and cut into long strips

1 red bell pepper, seeded and cut into long strips

1 orange bell pepper, seeded and cut into long strips

2 Roma tomatoes, seeded and diced

1 teaspoon Italian flat-leaf parsley, minced

1 cup boiling water

2 tablespoons balsamic vinegar mixed with 1 tablespoon extra-virgin olive oil

Salt and pepper to taste

In a medium saucepan sauté onion, garlic, and carrot in 3 tablespoons olive oil until the vegetables are coated with oil. Add the peppers, tomatoes, and parsley to the hot onion mixture. Pour in 1 cup boiling water and reduce the heat to a simmer. Cook until the peppers are very soft; approximately 30 minutes.

Add mixture to large serving bowl and cool to room temperature.

Toss with balsamic vinegar and olive oil. Taste and add kosher salt and fresh ground black pepper if needed.

190 calories | 10.33 g fat, 1.41 g saturated fat | 21.36 g carbohydrate | 2.9 g protein | 24 mg sodium | 1.75 g fiber

The Vitamin C Brigade

Peppers, tomatoes, onions, and parsley are packed with fiber as well as vitamin C, a powerful antioxidant that promotes a healthy liver.

Chapter 14

10-Day Gallbladder Detox

MANY PEOPLE THINK THE GALLBLADDER IS AN INSIGNIFICANT and dispensable organ. While it's true that you can survive without your gallbladder, once it's removed, your body must work harder to digest fats and remove cholesterol from the body. Having your gallbladder removed because you've been eating too much saturated fat and cholesterol (which creates gallstones) is like removing the engine from your car because you've been using the wrong kind of gas. The 10-Day Gallbladder Detox gives your gallbladder the "fuel" it needs to restore balance and prevent gallstones.

Your Gallbladder's Job

The gallbladder is a small, hollow, pear-shaped organ that stores and concentrates bile, an essential liquid for digestion. Bile, which is continually secreted by the liver and stored in the gallbladder, emulsifies fats and neutralizes the acids in foods that are partly digested.

When you consume too much saturated fat, substances in bile crystallize in the gallbladder and form gallstones, or small, hard substances that may be as small as a grain of sand or as large as a golf ball, called gallstones.

> **Food for Thought**
>
> *Gallstones are very common, affecting about one in twelve Americans. Gallstones are most common in people over age forty, especially women and people who are obese. Many people have "silent" gallstones that produce no symptoms. Once gallstones make their presence known, however, there's nothing silent about them. Symptoms range from indigestion and nausea to severe pain in the upper right abdomen.*

Small gallstones often pass from the body on their own, but large gallstones that cause serious blockage may require surgical removal. In some cases, the entire gallbladder must be removed. Every year, about 750,000 Americans have their gallbladder removed.

Your liver and gallbladder were designed to work together to digest fats. When your gallbladder is removed, your liver must work harder to digest fats. If you continue to eat a diet high in saturated fats and low in fiber, you may have a higher risk of developing heart disease and stroke.

How to Eat to Restore Balance

- Cleanse your gallbladder by going on a vegetarian or vegan diet to reduce your intake of cholesterol.
- Drink at least eight glasses of water a day to facilitate digestion and dilute toxic substances in food.
- Substitute heart-healthy plant-based oils like canola oil, olive oil, and sesame oil for butter, which contains saturated fat and cholesterol, and margarine, which contains dangerous trans fats.
- Replace fatty meats like burgers and steak with cold-water fish that is high in omega-3 fatty acids, including tuna, herring, mackerel, trout, and halibut.
- Eliminate processed and refined foods from your diet. They are high in saturated fats, trans fats, and cholesterol.
- Consume "cleansing" vegetable juices made from beets, beet greens, cucumbers, celery, and carrots.
- Eat plenty of fresh garlic, which has a cleansing effect on the liver.
- Drink lemon diluted with warm water in the morning to help cleanse the gallbladder
- Eat cruciferous veggies, including cabbage, kale, Brussels sprouts, and broccoli. They are high in fiber and help cleanse the gallbladder by promoting regularity.
- Consume eggs in moderation. Consuming too many eggs may aggravate gallbladder disease.
- Don't avoid fats entirely. Fat-free and low-fat diets can also cause gallstones, so consume heart-healthy oils in moderation.

As well as cleansing your gallbladder, this diet will help you lower your LDL "bad" cholesterol, lose weight, and reduce your risk of heart disease and stroke. Other diets in this book that will help you reduce your intake of cholesterol and saturated fats and improve the health of your gallbladder include the 3-Day Fruit Fast, the 10-Day Cholesterol Flush, the 10-Day Raw Foods Detox, the 15-Day Vegan Detox, and the 15-Day Mediterranean Detox.

Meal Plans for 10-Day Gallbladder Detox

To prevent gallstones, don't skip meals and eat on a regular schedule. Also, don't avoid fat altogether, as this can cause the gallbladder to get out of shape. Just stick to healthy fats, like those found in nuts and seeds. Bonus: A Harvard study showed that eating nuts and seeds lowered the incidence of gallbladder problems in women!

Breakfast

1 serving Baked Oatmeal with Bananas (page 220)
8 ounces Orange Beet Juice (page 11)
Herbal Tea or Coffee

Lunch

2 cups Baby Spring Greens with 3 ounces Seared Tuna and Balsamic Vinaigrette
1 slice Garlic Bread
Herbal Tea

Dinner

1 cup Ratatouille over ½ cup Couscous
½ cup Steamed Broccoli with Lemon
Tropical Sherbet
Herbal Tea

Day 1

Breakfast

Blueberry Crepes
Canadian Bacon
Herbal Tea or Coffee

Lunch

1 small Spinach Calzone
1 cup Chicken and Wild Rice Soup
Herbal Tea

Dinner

1 serving Linguine with Lemon and Artichokes (page 221)
½ cup Sliced Tomatoes with Olive Oil and Cracked Black Pepper
1 medium Slice French Bread
Homemade Apple Crisp

Day 2

Breakfast

¾ cup Muesli with Craisins and Fresh Peaches
1 cup Low-Fat Milk or Soy Milk
Herbal Tea

Lunch

8 ounces Carrot Celery Cucumber Juice
1 Pita Bread with Hummus, Chopped Romaine, and Tomatoes
Herbal Tea

Dinner

4 ounces Roasted Beef Tenderloin
½ cup Rice with Raisins (page 222)
½ cup Sautéed Swiss Chard
1 cup Garden Salad
¾ cup Blackberries with Vanilla Yogurt
Herbal Tea

Day 3

Meal Plans for 10-Day Gallbladder Detox

Day 4

Breakfast
2 Scrambled Egg Tacos with Fresh Salsa in Corn Tortillas
1 cup Watermelon and Cantaloupe Chunks
Herbal Tea

Lunch
1 medium Baked Potato Topped with Steamed Broccoli and Low-Fat Cheddar
1 cup Tomato and Red Onion Salad with Italian Dressing
Herbal Tea

Dinner
1 serving Ginger-Glazed Salmon (page 223)
½ cup Brown Rice Pilaf
½ cup Roasted Asparagus
1 cup Baby Spring Greens with Lemon and Olive Oil
2 Broiled Peach Halves with Low-Fat Vanilla Ice Cream
Herbal Tea

Day 5

Breakfast
1 slice Whole Wheat Toast with Avocado
8 ounces Orange Beet Greens Juice
Herbal Tea

Lunch
1 serving Italian Pasta Salad (page 224)
1 cup Mixed Fruit with Chopped Walnuts
Herbal Tea

Dinner
4 ounces Garlic-Roasted Chicken
½ cup Mashed Potatoes
½ cup Steamed Broccoli
1 cup Garden Salad
1 Whole Wheat Dinner Roll
Herbal Tea

Day 6

Breakfast
1 cup Steel-Cut Oatmeal with Dates and Nuts
1 cup Low-Fat Milk or Soy Milk
2 slices Turkey Bacon
Herbal Tea

Lunch
1 cup Homemade Tomato Soup
1 small Garlic Parmesan Toasted Baguette
1 cup Garden Salad with Low-Fat Dressing
Herbal Tea

Dinner
4 ounces Lentil Loaf (page 31)
½ cup Roasted Green Beans (page 225)
½ cup Mashed Sweet Potato
½ cup Rice with Parsley
½ cup Chocolate Pudding with Sliced Bananas
Herbal Tea

Day 7

Breakfast
½ cup Granola
1 cup Yogurt
½ cup Fruit Salad
Herbal Tea

Lunch
1 Avocado Sprout Wrap with Tomatoes
1 serving Five-Bean Salad (page 226)
Herbal Tea

Dinner
1 cup Chicken and Rice Casserole with Green Chilies and Low-Fat Cheese
½ cup Pan-Seared Zucchini with Garlic
1 cup Spring Greens Salad
½ cup Rainbow Sherbet
Herbal Tea

Meal Plans for 10-Day Gallbladder Detox

Breakfast

1 Baked Apple Stuffed with
  Nuts and Raisins (page
  227)
1 cup Yogurt
1 slice Whole Wheat Toast
Herbal Tea

Lunch

1 cup Minestrone Soup (see
  page 60)
½ Egg Salad Sandwich with
  Low-Fat Mayo on Whole-
  Grain Bread
½ cup Celery and Carrot
  Sticks
Herbal Tea

Dinner

4 ounces Grilled Halibut
1 cup Chunky Greek Salad
  (page 56)
½ cup Sautéed Spinach with
  Mushrooms
½ cup Boiled Red Potatoes
  with Olive Oil
1 Wedge Angel Food Cake
  with Sliced Strawberries and
  Low-Fat Whipped Topping
Herbal Tea

Day 8

Breakfast

1 medium Bagel with Light
  Cream Cheese
2 slices Turkey Bacon
6 ounces Apple Juice
Herbal Tea

Lunch

1 wedge Asparagus Fritatta
1 cup Baby Spring Greens
  with Lemon and Olive Oil
1 sliced Orange
Herbal Tea

Dinner

4 ounces Turkey Medallions
1 serving Cranberry Nut Rice
  Salad (page 228)
1 cup Roasted Acorn Squash
¾ cup Peach Crisp
Herbal Tea

Day 9

Breakfast

8 ounces Apple Celery Juice
1 cup Oatmeal with Dried
  Fruit and Low-Fat Milk or
  Soy Milk
Herbal Tea

Lunch

½ cup Middle-Eastern
  Roasted Eggplant Tahini
  Dip (baba ghanoush)
1 Whole Wheat Pita Bread
1 cup Curry-Spiced Carrot
  Raisin Salad
Herbal Tea

Dinner

1 cup Pasta with Pan-Seared
  Scallops with Garlic,
  Shrimp, Olive Oil, and
  Lemon Juice
1 cup Spinach Salad with
  Mushrooms and Radishes
1 cup Low-Fat Milk or Soy
  Milk
1 serving Blackberry Crisp
  (page 228)

Day 10

Recipes for 10-Day Gallbladder Detox

Baked Oatmeal with Bananas

Serves: 6

INGREDIENTS

2 cups cooked oatmeal

2 bananas, sliced

2 eggs, beaten

1 cup low-fat cottage cheese

¾ cup skim milk or half-and-half

1 teaspoon cinnamon

½ teaspoon nutmeg

½ teaspoon kosher salt

Pure maple syrup

Blend oatmeal, bananas, eggs, cottage cheese, milk, cinnamon, nutmeg, and salt.

Pour into an ovenproof dish sprayed with cooking spray and bake at 350°F for 40 minutes or until oatmeal is puffed up.

Serve with pure maple syrup.

180 calories | 4.56 g fat, 1.35 g saturated fat | 21.66 g carbohydrate | 12.98 g protein | 387 mg sodium | .45 g fiber

Why Is Oatmeal a Better Wake-Up Call for Your Gallbladder Than Captain Crunch?

Low in fat and high in fiber, oatmeal helps cleanse your intestinal tract, which in turn improves the health of your gallbladder. Sugary breakfast cereals are loaded with refined flours, sugars, and salt, all of which may contribute to the formation of gallstones.

Recipes for 10-Day Gallbladder Detox

Linguine with Lemons and Artichokes

Serves: 2

INGREDIENTS

6 ounces linguine

1 cup green onion, sliced thin

1 tablespoon olive oil

8 ounces canned artichoke hearts, drained and rinsed

1 cup low-sodium chicken broth

½ cup dry white wine

¼ cup skim milk

1 teaspoon lemon zest

1 lemon cut into wedges

3 tablespoons Italian flat-leaf parsley, minced

Cook linguine in boiling water. Drain.

Sauté onions in olive oil. Add artichoke hearts, chicken broth, wine, milk, and lemon zest.

Stir until boiling. Sauce will slightly thicken.

Place artichoke sauce over linguine in warm bowls. Garnish with parsley and lemon wedges.

528 calories | 13.42 g fat, 3.66 g saturated fat | 88.28 g carbohydrate | 18.43 g protein | 135 mg sodium | 1.77 g fiber

Why Are Artichokes a Superfood for Your Gallbladder?

Artichokes are a great source of unsaturated fat, fiber, and vitamin C, all of which help cleanse and support the liver, which in turn promotes a healthy gallbladder.

Rice with Raisins

Serves: 4

INGREDIENTS

1 cup white onion, chopped

1½ cups white rice

2 tablespoons unsalted butter

2 cups reduced-sodium beef broth

1 cup water

1 teaspoon cinnamon

1 teaspoon nutmeg

1 teaspoon ground ginger

2 teaspoons ground cloves

¾ cup golden raisins

Sauté onion and rice in butter until onion is soft.

Add beef broth, water, and spices and bring to a boil.

Reduce heat and simmer until rice is cooked (approximately 30 minutes).

Stir in raisins.

Serve immediately.

439 calories | 6.88 g fat, 3.95 g saturated fat | 86.45 g carbohydrate | 7.83 g protein | 51 mg sodium | 1.16 g fiber

How Do Raisins Prevent Gallstones?

Raisins are packed with fiber to help prevent constipation, which may lead to the formation of gallstones.

Ginger-Glazed Salmon

Serves: 2

INGREDIENTS

3 tablespoons extra-virgin olive oil

2 tablespoons fresh gingerroot, peeled, grated

⅛ cup low-sodium soy sauce

1 tablespoon sugar

1 teaspoon sake

½ teaspoon sesame oil

1 orange, zest and juice

10 ounces wild salmon, rinsed, trimmed of any fat

How Can Salmon Help Your Gallbladder?

To keep gallbladder problems in check, replace fatty meats with cold-water fish like salmon, which is high in omega-3 fatty acids and protein.

Combine olive oil, ginger, soy sauce, sugar, sake, sesame oil, juice, and zest.

Pour mixture over salmon in a shallow baking dish and marinate for 1–2 hours.

Sauté salmon in olive oil over high heat. The salmon will take on a dark caramelized appearance. Turn over and finish cooking. Lower the heat if necessary.

453 calories | 32 g fat, 4.8 g saturated fat | 10.21 g carbohydrate | 30.48 g protein | 549 mg sodium | .04 g fiber

Italian Pasta Salad

Serves: 4

INGREDIENTS

4 Roma tomatoes, seeded, diced

4 green onions, sliced

1 cucumber, peeled and diced

1 red bell pepper, diced

1 zucchini, diced

¼ cup green olives, sliced

2 pepperoncinis, diced (juice reserved)

1 cup artichoke hearts, canned in water, quartered

2 cups whole wheat pasta, cooked according to package directions

Salt and fresh ground black pepper to taste

¾ cup balsamic vinegar

½ cup extra-virgin olive oil

2 tablespoons fresh basil, minced

1 tablespoon brown sugar

⅓ cup Parmigiano-Reggiano cheese, grated

2 tablespoons pine nuts, toasted

Combine tomatoes, green onion, cucumber, red pepper, zucchini, green olives, pepperoncinis, artichoke hearts, and pasta. Season to taste with salt and freshly ground black pepper.

To make salad dressing combine balsamic vinegar, olive oil, reserved pepperoncini juice, basil, and brown sugar.

Pour salad dressing over pasta and vegetables.

Refrigerate for 2 or more hours.

Serve salad with Parmigiano-Reggiano cheese and pine nuts sprinkled on top.

234 calories | 6.61 g fat, 2.08 g saturated fat | 34.19 g carbohydrate | 9.4 g protein | 370 mg sodium | 2.46 g fiber

Why Do Italians Have Fewer Gallstones Than Americans?

This authentic Italian recipe is packed with a cornucopia of vegetables that supply a rainbow of nutrients that support your liver and gallbladder, including fiber and vitamin C.

Roasted Green Beans

Serves: 2

INGREDIENTS

½ medium onion, sliced

2 cloves garlic, sliced

2 tablespoons balsamic vinegar

1 teaspoon lemon zest

3 tablespoons extra-virgin olive oil

Salt and pepper to taste

10 ounces fresh green beans, trimmed

Mix onion, garlic, balsamic vinegar, lemon zest, olive oil, and salt and pepper together in a small bowl.

Preheat oven to 425°F.

Place green beans in a large bowl and pour mixture over them.

Line a baking sheet with foil and spray with pan spray.

Bake beans 20–25 minutes or until golden brown.

Serve immediately.

242 calories | 19.69 g fat, 2.67 g saturated fat | 13.55 g carbohydrate | 2.61 g protein | 638 mg sodium | 1.54 g fiber

Five-Bean Salad

Serves: 6

INGREDIENTS

½ pound green beans, trimmed

8 ounces low-sodium garbanzo beans, drained and rinsed

8 ounces no-salt kidney beans, drained and rinsed

8 ounces low-sodium white beans, drained and rinsed

8 ounces low-sodium black beans, drained and rinsed

1 medium onion, diced

1 tablespoon minced garlic

1 cup apple cider vinegar

¼ cup brown sugar

¼ cup olive oil

black pepper to taste

Blanch green beans by placing them in boiling water for 3 minutes and then directly into a bowl of ice water to stop the cooking.

Combine all beans plus onions and garlic in a large glass or nonreactive bowl.

Whisk vinegar, brown sugar, oil, and black pepper together.

Pour vinegar mixture over beans, cover, and refrigerate.

Let beans sit overnight if possible so that the flavors infuse.

314 calories | 11.79 g fat, 1.55 g saturated fat | 39.1 g carbohydrate | 12.87 g protein | 342 mg sodium | 3.23 g fiber

Why Are Beans a Healthier Choice?

Gallstones are often caused by consuming too much cholesterol, which is found in animal proteins. You can lower your cholesterol by eating more beans, a low-fat food that's packed with gallbladder-friendly plant protein and fiber.

Recipes for 10-Day Gallbladder Detox

Baked Apples Stuffed with Nuts and Raisins

Serves: 2

INGREDIENTS

2 large apples, such as Macintosh, Rome, or Granny Smith

2 teaspoons brown sugar

1 teaspoon cinnamon

2 teaspoons chopped walnuts

2 teaspoons raisins

1 tablespoon butter

Apples for a Healthy Gallbladder

Apples help cleanse the liver and colon, which improves the function of the gallbladder.

Preheat the oven to 350°F. Using a corer, remove the center portions of the apples, being careful not to cut through the bottom of the apple.

Form a cup with a double layer of aluminum foil, going ⅓ of the way up the apple. This will stabilize the apple when baking.

Mix together the brown sugar, cinnamon, walnuts, and raisins and stuff the mixture into the apples. Top each apple with 1 teaspoon of butter. Put 1 tablespoon of water into the aluminum foil cups.

Bake for 25 minutes or until the apples are soft when pricked with a fork.

Serve immediately.

296 calories | 11.85 g fat, 7 g saturated fat | 46.69 g carbohydrate | .58 g protein | 7 mg sodium | 4.53 g fiber

Recipes for 10-Day Gallbladder Detox

Cranberry Nut Rice Salad

Serves: 4

INGREDIENTS

2 teaspoons extra-virgin olive oil

1 garlic clove, peeled and minced

¼ cup almonds, chopped

1½ cups brown rice

1 teaspoon cumin

1½ cups low-sodium chicken broth

1 cup water

½ cup dried cranberries

2 tablespoons Italian parsley, minced

Heat olive oil in sauce pan over medium heat. Sauté garlic for 30 seconds. Add almonds and cook for another 30 seconds. Add brown rice and cumin, stirring constantly. Add broth and water and bring to a boil. Reduce heat to a simmer and cook until rice is done, approximately 45 minutes.

Remove from heat and add craisins and parsley.

401 calories | 10 g fat, 1.23 g saturated fat | 66.64 g carbohydrate | 8.8 g protein | 175 mg sodium | 2.48 g fiber

Blackberry Crisp

Serves: 8

INGREDIENTS

3 cups blackberries

¾ cup flour

¾ cup sugar

½ teaspoon salt

1 teaspoon cinnamon

½ teaspoon ground nutmeg

1 teaspoon almond extract

8 tablespoons unsalted butter, cut into small cubes

Preheat oven to 375°F.

Using a food processor, combine the dry ingredients, almond extract, and the cubes of butter. Pulse until a crumb mixture forms. Do not overmix.

Place the blackberries in a glass 8" × 8" baking dish coated with pan spray.

Place the crumb topping on the blackberries and bake 45 minutes or until hot and bubbly.

250 calories | 11.45 g fat, 6.94 g saturated fat | 35 g carbohydrate | 1.74 g protein | 142 mg sodium | 2.36 g fiber

Chapter 15

5-Day Intestinal Detox

WHEN YOU EAT SOMETHING, YOUR INTESTINES GET BUSY absorbing fat-soluble vitamins, cholesterol, fat, proteins, carbohydrates, and bile salts. Your small intestines absorb the majority of nutrients from your food, while the large intestine forms stool and absorbs water, as well as electrolytes and mineral salts that regulate fluid balance. Consuming too much sugar, fried foods, spoiled foods, caffeine, and/or prescription drugs may stimulate the formation of toxic secretions on the intestinal wall, which in turn may hinder your body's ability to absorb nutrients and eliminate waste products.

Inside Your Intestine

If you consume the Standard American Diet (SAD), your intestinal health may be in equally sad shape because it's probably high in processed and refined foods that are loaded with sugar, saturated fat, cholesterol, trans fats, and caffeine.

All these foods contribute to constipation because they are low in fiber and healthy, unsaturated fats such as nuts, seeds, and plant-based oils, which help soften the stool and add bulk to promote elimination. Various factors can cause constipation, including:

Processed foods that are made with refined white flour, white rice, and white sugar, including cookies, pastries, crackers, and breads where the fiber has been removed.

Snack foods that are high in saturated fats, trans fats, and cholesterol, including pizza, ice cream, cheese, hamburgers, hot dogs, French fries, milk shakes, and potato chips.

Foods that are high in sugar, caffeine, or alcohol, including coffee, tea, beer, wine, fruit drinks, and cola drinks.

Not eating enough fiber. Psyllium, bran, and other bulking supplements can help increase the volume of stools and promote regularity.

Taking too much calcium supplementation may cause constipation.

Stress, tension, and worry. Stress can slow things down in your digestive tract and result in constipation, or speed them up and result in nausea, vomiting, and diarrhea. You can help alleviate stress by taking a walk; doing yoga, deep breathing, or meditation; or taking a hot bath with Epsom salts.

Many prescription drugs cause constipation. If the manufacturer says the drug may cause constipation, increase your intake of fiber; reduce your intake of sugar, unhealthy fats, white flour products, junk food, and fast food; and get more daily exercise.

Traveling, flying, or anything that disrupts your internal rhythms can also result in constipation. The low humidity in airplanes may rob your body of needed moisture and lead to dehydration, which can cause constipation.

Not drinking enough water. You should drink from 8 to 10 glasses of water daily for internal lubrication and to prevent constipation. If you don't like drinking plain water, try consuming additional water in herbal teas or vitamin waters.

Vitamin deficiencies, especially a lack of C and B complex, may cause constipation.

Fiber to the Rescue

Eating lots of fiber helps foods move through your intestinal tract quickly and efficiently and prevents constipation, hemorrhoids, high cholesterol, high blood sugar, obesity, colon cancer, and heart disease. Unfortunately, most Americans consume just 5 to 14 grams of fiber daily, as opposed to the 24 to 38 grams needed for healthy digestion.

Many fruits and vegetables help lubricate your intestines and promote regularity. To prevent constipation, make sure you consume the following foods on a regular basis.

Fruits, especially apples, bananas, blueberries, figs, grapefruit, peaches, pears, raspberries, and strawberries.

Vegetables, especially avocadoes, cabbage, carrots, cauliflower, corn, green beans, kale, peas, potatoes, spinach, sweet potatoes, and winter squash.

Cereals and grains, especially bran, oats, brown rice, and whole wheat pasta.

All types of **beans, nuts, and seeds.**

Yogurt—the active-culture in yogurt helps repopulate your digestive system with organisms that aid in breaking down food, while the acidophilus in yogurt encourages healthy bacterial growth.

Meal Plans for 5-Day Intestinal Detox

In addition to the foods suggested here, you may want to work yogurt (with live or active cultures), fermented foods (sauerkraut, for example), and oatmeal (not instant!) into your regular rotation to keep your intestines in good health. Adding a probiotic to the mix will promote the growth of beneficial bacteria and keep balance in your intestines.

Breakfast

1 Whole Wheat English Muffin with Peanut Butter
1 cup Yogurt with Fresh Peaches and Nuts
Herbal Tea

Lunch

1 serving Broccoli Soup (page 233)
1 serving Mixed Greens with Berries and Orange Vinaigrette (page 234)
1 slice Whole Wheat Bread, Toasted
Herbal Tea

Dinner

1 wedge Artichoke and Red Pepper Frittata
½ cup Italian Sautéed Vegetables
1 slice Whole Wheat Garlic Bread
½ cup Lemon Sorbet
Herbal Tea

Breakfast

1 cup Oatmeal with Raisins, Nuts and Cinnamon
1 cup Low-Fat Milk or Soy Milk
Herbal Tea

Lunch

2 cups Tuna Niçoise Salad with Lemon Juice and Olive Oil
1 small Whole Wheat Baguette
Herbal Tea

Dinner

1 serving Pasta, Tomatoes, and Basil (page 235)
1 cup Garden Salad
½ cup Broiled Figs with Honeyed Yogurt
Herbal Tea

Breakfast

½ cup Cold Bran Cereal with Bananas
1 cup Low-Fat Milk or Soy Milk
1 cup Cantaloupe Chunks and Blueberries
Herbal Tea

Lunch

1 serving Hot Artichoke and Roasted Red Pepper Dip (page 236)
1 serving Low-Sodium Wheat Thin-Type Crackers
½ cup Red Cabbage and Green Apple Coleslaw with Raisins and Apple Cider Vinaigrette
Herbal Tea

Dinner

1 serving Black Bean Soup (page 237)
1 corn Muffin
1 cup Garden Salad
¾ cup Vanilla Frozen Yogurt with Raspberries
Herbal Tea

Meal Plans for 5-Day Intestinal Detox

Breakfast

1 Berry Muffin (page 238)
2 ounces Canadian Bacon
½ cup Mixed Fruit with a
    Dollop of Yogurt
Herbal Tea

Lunch

1 cup Stir-Fried Broccoli,
    Carrots, Summer Squash,
    Peppers, Snow Peas, and
    Tofu
½ cup Brown Rice
½ cup Red Grapes
Herbal Tea

Dinner

1 Veggie Burger with Barbe-
    cue Sauce, Lettuce, Tomato,
    and Whole Wheat Bun
Roasted Potatoes (page 239)
½ cup Grilled Pineapple with
    Coconut Sorbet
Herbal Tea

Breakfast

1 cup Steel-Cut Oats with
    Dates and Nuts
1 cup Low-Fat Milk or Soy
    Milk
1 sliced Apple with Peanut
    Butter
Herbal Tea

Lunch

6-inch Vegetable Pizza with
    Low-Fat Cheese on Whole
    Wheat Crust
1 cup Baby Spring Greens
    Salad
Herbal Tea

Dinner

1 serving Three-Bean Chili
    (page 240)
1 serving Southwestern
    Brown Rice (page 241)
1 cup Corn Salad with Red
    Bell Pepper, Cucumber,
    Sweet Onion, Cilantro,
    Lime Juice, and Olive Oil
1 serving Baked Pears with
    Goat Cheese and Pecans
    (page 242)
Herbal Tea

Recipes for 5-Day Intestinal Detox

Broccoli Soup

Serves: 4

INGREDIENTS

3 tablespoons unsalted butter

3 tablespoons flour

2 tablespoons olive oil

1½ pounds broccoli, stems and florets

1 onion, diced

2 cloves garlic, minced

1 teaspoon dried tarragon

2 cups low-sodium, low-fat chicken broth

1 cup skim milk

½ cup low-fat Cheddar cheese, grated

Natural Lubricants

Cruciferous veggies like broccoli add bulk to your stool and also help lubricate your intestines, which in turn promotes healthy elimination.

Mix the butter and flour together with your hands in a small bowl. Form into small balls and refrigerate. This mixture is a cold roux and will serve as the thickening agent for the soup.

Place olive oil in large pot. Add broccoli stems and onion and sauté until onion is soft. Add garlic and tarragon and stir for 30 seconds. Add chicken broth and bring mixture to boil, reduce heat and simmer until broccoli is soft.

Stir in roux and cook for at least 10 minutes to remove any trace of flour taste.

Stir in broccoli florets. Cook for 5 minutes.

Add skim milk and cheese and stir well until cheese is melted.

Serve in warm bowls.

342 calories | 19 g fat, 7.5 g saturated fat | 26 g carbohydrate | 15.28 g protein | 179 mg sodium | 9 g fiber

Recipes for 5-Day Intestinal Detox

Mixed Greens with Berries and Orange Vinaigrette

Serves: 2

INGREDIENTS

1 cup mixed greens

1 cup fresh raspberries

1 cup fresh strawberries, sliced

¼ cup white wine vinegar

1 orange, juice and zest

1 teaspoon coarse-grain mustard

¼ cup extra-virgin olive oil

Salt and pepper to taste

⅛ cup walnut halves, toasted

Rinse salad greens and berries and dry well.

Whisk vinegar, orange juice, and zest with mustard and olive oil until thick. Season with salt and pepper to taste.

Toss greens with salad dressing.

Place on cold salad plate and top with berries and walnuts.

383 calories | 32 g fat, 4 g saturated fat | 19.74 g carbohydrate | 3.12 g protein | 41 mg sodium | 8 g fiber

The Salad That Keeps Giving

Strawberries, raspberries, and leafy greens are all abundant in fiber and help flush your colon to promote a healthy intestinal tract. The olive oil and walnuts in this recipe provide healthy omega-3 fatty acids that lubricate the intestinal tract and facilitate elimination.

Recipes for 5-Day Intestinal Detox

Pasta, Tomatoes, and Beans

Serves: 4

INGREDIENTS

⅛ cup extra-virgin olive oil

1 clove garlic, minced

2 tomatoes, seeded and diced

2 cups white beans, soaked overnight and cooked

1½ cups broccoli, steamed

Salt and pepper to taste

Dried Italian seasoning, to taste

¾ pound whole wheat pasta, cooked

¼ cup Parmesan cheese, grated

Heat olive oil in large frying pan over medium heat. Add the garlic and tomatoes and let sauté for 2–3 minutes. Lower the heat and add beans and broccoli. Cook for 5 minutes.

Season to taste with salt, pepper, and Italian seasoning.

Place pasta in bowls and ladle bean and broccoli mixture over the top. Add grated Parmesan cheese and serve immediately.

Why This Is the Perfect Pasta Dish

This healthy take on pasta provides lots of fiber from beans, whole wheat pasta, and broccoli, plus just enough polyunsaturated fats from olive oil to keep things moving along.

579 calories | 11.99 g fat, 2.65 g saturated fat | 93.82 g carbohydrate | 23.91 g protein | 378 mg sodium | 6 g fiber

Recipes for 5-Day Intestinal Detox

Hot Artichoke and Roasted Red Pepper Dip

Serves: 8

INGREDIENTS

1 leek, cleaned and diced

2 teaspoons unsalted butter

4 large artichokes, steamed, hearts removed and coarsely chopped

½ cup Parmesan cheese, grated

1 cup roasted red pepper, chopped

¾ cup light mayonnaise

Freshly ground black pepper to taste

10 ounces low-sodium Wheat Thins-type crackers

Sauté leek in medium skillet in unsalted butter until it is light brown. Remove from heat. Stir in artichoke hearts, cheese, roasted red peppers, mayonnaise, and black pepper.

Spray a 9-inch glass pie plate with pan spray and heat oven to 350°F. Place dip mixture into pie plate.

Bake uncovered for 20–25 minutes or until hot and bubbly. Serve with crackers.

305 calories | 14.2 g fat, 5.38 g saturated fat | 37.12 g carbohydrate | 7.27 g protein | 373 mg sodium | 7.59 g fiber

How Does Fiber Help Your Colon?

Studies show that consuming at least 25 grams of fiber every day may help prevent colon cancer. The artichokes, leeks, and red peppers in this recipe will give you a good head start on your daily quota of fiber.

Black Bean Soup

Serves: 4

INGREDIENTS

2 cups dried black beans

4½ cups water

1 onion, diced

1 carrot, peeled and diced

5 sprigs fresh thyme

3 cloves garlic, minced

1 bay leaf

2 teaspoons ground cumin

2 cups reduced-sodium, low-fat chicken broth

Salt and pepper to taste

¼ cup chopped cilantro

½ cup red onion, diced

Cover beans with cold water and soak overnight. Drain and pour into a large Dutch oven. Add 4½ cups water, onion, carrots, thyme, garlic, bay leaf, cumin and broth.

Simmer for 1 hour. Taste and season with salt and pepper.

Ladle into warm bowls and top with chopped cilantro and chopped onion.

Serve immediately.

---

393 calories | 2.21 g fat, .39 g saturated fat | 69.77 g carbohydrate | 23.42 g protein | 52 mg sodium | 6 g fiber

Beans for Bulk

Beans are an excellent source of low-fat, no-cholesterol fiber and protein. The fiber in beans adds bulk to your stool and helps keeps you regular without overloading you with the fat and cholesterol found in animal protein.

Recipes for 5-Day Intestinal Detox

Berry Muffins

Serves: 12

INGREDIENTS

½ cup oats

1 tablespoon lemon juice

½ cup skim milk

¾ cup whole wheat flour

¾ cup all-purpose flour

1 teaspoon baking powder

½ teaspoon baking soda

1 teaspoon ground cinnamon

1/2 teaspoon salt

1 orange, zest

½ cup granulated sugar

¼ cup canola oil

1 egg

1 cup fresh blueberries

1 cup fresh raspberries

Preheat oven to 400°F. Prepare muffin pans by lining them with cupcake papers.

Stir oats, lemon juice, and milk together in a small bowl and let sit for 5 minutes.

Combine flour, baking powder, baking soda, cinnamon, and salt. Set aside.

Grate rind (zest) from orange and add to a large bowl. Whisk in sugar, oil, and egg until mixture is combined. Add oatmeal mixture and flour. Do not overmix.

Fold in berries.

Spoon muffin batter into tins and bake for 15 minutes or until a tester comes out clean.

Berries Get Things Moving

The blueberries, raspberries, and oats in this recipe contain tons of fiber, which bulks up the stool, and facilitates elimination.

192 calories | 5.94 g fat, .6 g saturated fat | 30.97 g carbohydrate | 3.74 g protein | 126 mg sodium | 4 g fiber

Roasted Potatoes

Serves: 2

INGREDIENTS

2 russet potatoes, scrubbed, not peeled

1 teaspoon garlic, minced

1 tablespoon dried rosemary, crumbled

¼ teaspoon kosher salt and freshly ground black pepper

¼ cup extra-virgin olive oil

1 tablespoon grated Parmesan cheese

Hold the Fries!

Roasted potatoes provide lots of colon-friendly fiber without the colon-unfriendly saturated fats and cholesterol found in fast-food French fries.

Cut potatoes into French fry shapes. Place in large mixing bowl.

Combine oil, garlic, and rosemary in small bowl and add to the potato mixture.

Toss potatoes to ensure that they are well coated.

Line a baking sheet with foil and spray with pan spray.

Place potatoes on baking sheet and sprinkle with salt and pepper.

Bake in 400°F oven for 30–40 minutes or until brown and slightly crispy.

Sprinkle with Parmesan cheese immediately after removing from oven.

438 calories | 28.56 g fat, 4.22 g saturated fat | 29.8 g carbohydrate | 5.55 g protein | 352 mg sodium | 4 g fiber

Three-Bean Chili

Serves: 8

INGREDIENTS

3 tablespoons extra-virgin olive oil

1 onion, diced

2 cloves garlic, minced

1 (28–ounce) can whole tomatoes

1 (14½-ounce) can diced tomatoes

2 cups kidney beans, soaked overnight and cooked

2 cups black beans, soaked overnight and cooked

1 cup lima beans, soaked overnight and cooked

3 tablespoons chili powder

1 teaspoon dried basil

1 teaspoon dried oregano

1 teaspoon cumin

Salt and pepper to taste

Heat oil in large Dutch oven. Sauté onion until soft and translucent. Add garlic and sauté for 30 seconds.

Stir in tomatoes, beans, and seasoning and bring to a boil. Reduce heat to a simmer and cook for 1 hour on low heat.

Taste for seasoning, adjust if necessary.

Serve in warm bowls.

454 calories | 7.5 g fat, 1.4 g saturated fat | 71.47 g carbohydrate | 33.43 g protein | 285 mg sodium | 8 g fiber

Where's the Beef?

Beans, beans, and more beans provide a spicy and fiber-ific alternative to greasy meat chili, which is loaded with saturated fats and cholesterol, and which can cause constipation.

Southwestern Brown Rice

Serves: 4

INGREDIENTS

1 tablespoon extra-virgin olive oil

½ white onion, diced

1 serrano chili, minced

1 teaspoon chili powder

2 cups cooked brown rice, kept warm

1 cup black beans, drained and rinsed

1 cup frozen corn, thawed

4 ounces green chili, roasted and diced

2 tablespoons minced cilantro

Salt and pepper to taste

Heat oil in medium skillet over medium-low heat. Add onions and serrano and cook about 5 minutes or until onions are soft. Add chili powder and cook 1 additional minute.

Mix cooked rice, beans, corn, green chili, and cilantro into cooked onion mixture.

Taste and season with salt and pepper.

Serve immediately.

349 calories | 5.58 g fat, .61 g saturated fat | 65.11 g carbohydrate | 9.65 g protein | 256 mg sodium | 7 g fiber

Rice and Beans Are Nice to Your Colon

Brown rice, like beans, provides lots of fiber and protein without the saturated fat and cholesterol of animal protein that can clog up your intestines and arteries. Cilantro also helps stimulate intestinal motion. Brown rice and beans also form a complete protein.

Recipes for 5-Day Intestinal Detox

Baked Pears with Goat Cheese and Pecans

Serves: 2

INGREDIENTS

2 Bosc pears, cut in half and cored (do not peel)

½ cup honey

¼ cup high-quality balsamic vinegar

⅛ cup goat cheese

¼ cup toasted pecans, chopped small

The Stimulating Side of Pears and Pecans

Pears stimulate the intestinal tract and help promote healthy bowel movements, while pecans add bulk to the stool. Both are great for relieving constipation.

Spray a glass baking dish with pan spray.

Place pears, cut side down in the pan.

Whisk honey and balsamic vinegar together.

Bake pears for 20–30 minutes, or until soft when pierced.

Place pear cut side up on plate. Brush honey-balsamic mixture over the pear and top with goat cheese and pecans. Serve immediately.

485 calories | 12.7 g fat, 2.84 g saturated fat | 88.43 g carbohydrate | 4.28 g protein | 34 mg sodium | 6.12 g fiber

Index

About the Authors

Carole Jacobs is the former twenty-year senior editor, nutrition editor, and founding travel editor for *Shape* magazine and the former travel editor for *Living Fit*. Currently the fitness travel editor for *Travelgirl* magazine, she is also an award-winning freelance writer whose work has appeared in more than 250 national publications and has been syndicated by United Press Syndicate. Carole has authored/coauthored many books on nutrition, health, fitness, travel, and celebrities, including *Fat-Free and Fit*, *The Most Scenic Drives in America*, *The Everything® Juicing Book*, and *The Everything® Health Guide to Adult ADHD*.

Chef Patrice Johnson is a high-honors graduate of the California School of Culinary Arts in Pasadena, California, where she received a Le Cordon Bleu Culinary Degree. She is the a   :hool, and coau-
thor of *The Everythi*   r Personal Chef,
she specializes in ca   weekly dinners
for clients. In additic   children and
adults. Chef Patrice   roup exercise
instructor, and the o   in strength and
balance training for